For over 100 everyday ailments and health conditions Help is just a page away.

Help Yourself: You feel sick — but not sick enough to consult a doctor. Do you know how to help yourself? An irritating dry cough refuses to go away. Do you know how to treat yourself?

Safe and Natural Alternatives: When the doctor's prescription for your sinus or migraine or backache does not help, this book will. You will find sound advice to rejuvenate your heart and revitalise your body; to control dandruff and premature greying of hair; to detoxify your body of allergy causing chemicals; and to effectively cure indigestion and flatulence. All remedies given in the book are based on foods, herbs, vitamins, minerals and other natural substances likely to be available in your home.

Cures and Remedies that Work: Included in the book are remedies that have been successfully tested and filtered through centuries of experience and generations of use. Many of these have now been 'rediscovered' by modern scientific research. Reflecting the concern and tenor of the times, these remedies reject the fads associated with non-traditional healing and instead offer the best of natural healing backed with reliable medical guidance.

D0048451

The Author

H.K. Bakhru enjoys countrywide reputation as an expert naturopath and a writer on the subject. His well-researched articles on nature cure, health, and nutrition appear regularly in the media.

He began his career in the Indian Railways with a first class first postgraduate degree from Lucknow University. He retired, in 1984, as the Chief Public Relations Officer of the Central Railways, after 35 years of distinguished service in the Public Relations Organisation of the Indian Railways and the Railway Board.

A diploma holder in naturopathy, he is a member of the Nature Cure Practitioners' Guild in Mumbai. He has made extensive studies on naturopathy and herbalism. He spends his retired life propagating and practising nature cure and is always willing to offer advice to those who seek his help. His other books on nature cure, and nutrition are *Foods That Heal, Vitamins That Heal, Natural Home Remedies for Common Ailments, Conquering Diabetes Naturally, A Handbook of Natural Beauty, Nature Cure for Children's Diseases, Natural Health for the Elderly,* and *A Complete Handbook of Nature Cure.* He can be contacted at Flat 602, Building 9, Indus Cooperative Housing Society, MHADA HIG Complex, Oshiwara, Andheri (W), Mumbai-400 053. Tel: 2639 8779, Fax: 2639 8825. email: hkbakhru@hotmail.com

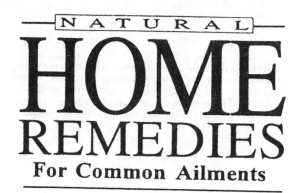

NATURAL
HOME
REMEDIES
For Common Ailments

H.K. Bakhru

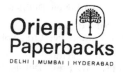

Orient
Paperbacks
DELHI | MUMBAI | HYDERABAD

www.orientpaperbacks.com

ISBN 13: 978-81-222-0179-6
ISBN 10: 81-222-0179-2

1st Published 1995
16th Printing 2011

Natural Home Remedies for Common Ailments

© H.K. Bakhru

Cover design by Vision Studio

Published by
Orient Paperbacks
(A division of Vision Books Pvt. Ltd.)
5A/8 Ansari Road, New Delhi-110 002

Printed in India at
Saurabh Printers Pvt. Ltd., Noida

Cover Printed at
Ravindra Printing Press, Delhi-110 006

Preface

Natural home remedies for common diseases is not a concept of the twentieth century. It is an age-old practice that has been passed down from one generation to the other, through trial and error. Home remedies are based on the knowledge that most natural foods like fruits, vegetables, cereal grains, seeds and nuts, as well as other natural substances, possess many medicinal virtues. These natural foods and substances have been tried and refined as natural cures in different countries. Research has proved many of these cures to be astonishingly effective. The living proof is that our ancestors—with the help of these cures—lived a happier, healthier, and longer life than the present generation.

Hippocrates, the Father of Medicine (460-357 B.C.), said: 'Nature cures, not the physician.'

He also advocated: 'Your food shall be your medicine.' This book is based on these maxims. It deals with over ninety diseases and their treatment through natural foods and other substances which are either available at home or easily obtainable from outside. None of the remedies prescribed here have potentially dangerous side-effects as do many modern drugs.

There are many books available on home remedies, but they are mostly based on traditional remedies. The distinctive feature of this book, however, is that besides mentioning the traditional remedies for various diseases, it prescribes nutritional treatments, including raw juice therapy, based on modern research. It also recommends time-tested natural methods of treatment and natural dietetics. This book may be therefore regarded as a handbook of natural home remedies, nature cure, and natural dietetics.

H.K. Bakhru

Contents

Acne

Acne is a common and chronic skin disease. It is an inflammatory condition of the sebaceous glands and hair follicles. The lesions are usually found on the skin of the face, neck, chest, and shoulders. Nearly six out of ten young people between the ages of twelve and twenty-four suffer from some degree of acne. The disease causes a great deal of embarrassment at an age when people tend to be sensitive about their personal appearance.

Causes and Symptoms

Acne is characterised by the presence of comedones or blackheads, pimples, small superficial sebaceous cysts, and scars. There are over half a dozen forms of acne, the most common being blackheads. The areas chiefly affected are the forehead, temples, cheeks, chin, chest, and back. In rare cases, almost the entire body may be covered with blackheads accompanied by extensive scarring.

All forms of acne have their origin in wrong eating habits, such as irregular hours of eating, excessive consumption of starch, sugar, fried and fatty foods. Chronic constipation is another cause of acne. If the bowels do not move properly, the waste matter is not eliminated as quickly as it should be and the bloodstream becomes surcharged with toxic matter. The extra efforts of the skin to eliminate excess waste result in acne and other forms of skin diseases. Other causes of this disorder are a devitalised condition of the skin resulting from unhygienic living habits, excessive use of tea, coffee, alcohol, or tobacco, and sedentary habits which lead to indigestion and general debility.

Remedies

Vitamins: Two vitamins, namely, niacin and vitamin A have been used successfully to treat acne. Vitamin therapy should comprise the intake of 100 mg niacin, three times daily, and 50,000 international units of vitamin A, three times daily. Vitamin E, 400 mg, should be taken once daily. This therapy should be continued for a month.

Zinc: Another effective remedy in the area of nutrition that seems to offer new promise of help for acne is zinc. It has shown dramatic results in some cases. Zinc should be taken in therapeutic doses of 50 mg three times a day. Zinc is available in tablet and in capsule form. In tablet form, it is available as Zinfet - 200 mg (Yash Pharma, Bombay). The patient can take a quarter tablet so as to get 50 mg of zinc. In capsule form, zinc is available as Ulseal– 220 mg (Tam Pharmaceuticals). One-fourth of the powder inside the capsule can be taken as a single dose. The patient can take a dose of 50 mg daily upto one month or till there is noticeable improvement and then reduce the dose to 25 mg.

Orange Peel: Orange peel has been found very effective in the local treatment of acne. Pounded well with water on a piece of stone, the peel should be applied to the affected areas.

Lemon: Lemon has also proved beneficial in reducing pimples and acne. Its juice should be applied regularly to obtain relief.

Garlic: Garlic has been used successfully in the treatment of acne. Pimples disappear without scars when rubbed with raw garlic several times a day. Even extremely persistent forms of acne, suffered by some adults, have been healed with this herb. The external use of garlic helps to clear the skin of spots, pimples and boils. The process is further helped by eating three pods of raw garlic once daily for a month to purify the blood stream, so as to secure a long-term clearance of the skin.

Coriander and Mint Juice: A teaspoon of coriander juice, mixed with a pinch of turmeric powder, is another effective home remedy for pimples and blackheads. The mixture should be applied to the face after thoroughly washing it every night before retiring. Mint juice can be used in a similar manner as coriander juice.

Fenugreek: Fenugreek is another useful remedy for acne. A paste made of the leaves of this vegetable, applied over the face every night before going to bed and washed with warm water in the morning, prevents pimples and blackheads.

Cucumber: Grated cucumber applied over the face, eyes, and neck for fifteen to twenty minutes has been found effective. It is the best tonic for the skin of the face. Its regular use prevents pimples and blackheads.

Dietary Considerations

To begin with, the patient should take only an 'all-fruit' diet for a week, taking three meals a day, of fresh juicy fruits, such as apples, pears, grapes, grapefruit, pineapples, and peaches. Only unsweetened lemon or plain water, either hot or cold, should be drunk and nothing else. After the one-week, all-fruit diet, the patient can gradually adopt a well-balanced diet with emphasis on raw foods, especially fresh fruit and vegetables, sprouted seeds, raw nuts, and wholegrain cereals, particularly millet and brown rice. Further short periods of the 'all-fruit' diet for three days or so may be necessary at a monthly interval till the skin's condition improves. Meats, sugar, strong tea or coffee, condiments, pickles, soft drinks, candies, ice cream, refined and processed foods should be avoided as far as possible.

Other Measures

During the initial one week 'all-fruit' diet, a warm-water enema should be taken daily to cleanse the bowels.

Hot fomentation should be applied locally to open up the pores and to bring out the waste matter. The affected parts should then be rinsed with cold water. The patient should take sun and air baths by exposing the whole body to the sun and air. A hot Epsom salts bath twice a week is beneficial in all cases of acne. This bath is prepared by adding 1 $\frac{1}{2}$ kg of Epsom salts to 60 litres of water having a temperature of about 37.8°C. The patient should remain in the bath tub for 25–35 minutes till he sweats freely. After the bath, the patient should cool off gradually.

Alcoholism

Alcohol Addiction

Alcoholism is a chronic disorder in which a person is unable to refrain from frequent and excessive consumption of alcohol.

Causes and Symptoms

Alcoholics have a puffy face with bloodshot eyes, hoarse voice and a rapid pulse. They are suspicious, irritable and over-emotional. Vomiting, delirium, impaired judgement, and disturbed sleep are some of the other symptoms that alcoholics suffer from. Excessive drinking damages the liver and gradually leads to cirrhosis. It also leads to disorders of the stomach and bowels. It can cause damage to the brain cells, and also affects the heart, which becomes weak and flabby.

Alcoholism starts with the individual taking an occasional drink. This gradually becomes a habit and leads to a state where the person cannot do without alcohol. Some people drink alcohol to enliven social gatherings under social pressure; for others, it is an escape from the responsibilities or stresses of life.

Remedies

Grapes: The most important home remedy for alcoholism is an exclusive diet, for a month or so, of grapes. Since this fruit contains the purest form of alcohol, it is an ideal yet healthy substitute for alcohol. Alcoholics should take three meals a day of fresh grapes at five-hourly intervals. The success of this treatment depends on the determination of the alcoholic to stop drinking.

Apples: Apples are another effective remedy for alcoholism. A generous intake of apples helps remove intoxication and reduces the craving for wines and other intoxicating liquors.

Dates: Dates are considered beneficial in the treatment of alcoholism. The patient should drink half a glass of water in which four or five dates have been rubbed together. This remedy should be taken twice daily for a month. It will bring definite relief.

Bitter Gourd: The juice of the leaves of bitter gourd is an antidote for alcohol intoxication. It is also useful for a liver damaged due to alcoholism. Three teaspoons of this juice, mixed with a glass of butter milk, should be taken every morning for a month.

Celery: The juice of raw celery has also been found useful in alcoholism. It exercises a sobering effect on the patient and is an antidote to alcohol. Half a glass of celery juice mixed with an equal quantity of water should be taken once daily for a month.

Dietary Considerations

The most effective way to treat alcoholism is to build up the body's nutritional integrity so as to prevent craving for stimulants like drinks. The patient should be put on a cleansing juice fast for at least ten days in the beginning.

During the juice fast, the patient will gradually feel less craving for alcohol. This is a good beginning towards breaking the drinking habit. After the initial fast of juices, the patient should take an optimum diet of vital nutrients consisting of wholegrain cereals, nuts, seeds and sprouts, fresh fruits, and vegetables.

It is advisable that at the beginning of the treatment, the patient is given a suitable substitute to relieve the craving if and when it occurs. The best substitute drink for alcohol is a glass of fresh fruit juice. The patient should drink juices and eat candy or other snacks if he feels a craving for a stimulant. All refined foods such as sugar, white rice, macaroni products, strong condiments, white flour, and meat should be avoided. The patient should eat several small meals a day in preference to two or three large ones.

Plenty of rest and outdoor physical exercises are also necessary.

Other Measures

The most important step towards breaking the 'alcohol habit' is the willingness of an alcoholic to do so. He must make a firm resolve to make a clean break at once, as giving up in stages is next to impossible.

During the first ten days of the 'juice fast', a warm-water enema should be taken everyday to cleanse the bowels. Smoking must be avoided as it increases the desire for alcohol. Plenty of rest and outdoor physical exercises are also necessary.

Allergies

Asthma, Rhinitis, Eczema[1]

The word 'allergy' means an altered or abnormal tissue reaction after exposure to an antigen (also called an 'allergen'). The allergic reaction occurs if the body tissues are sensitive to the allergen. The allergen may reach the tissues by direct contact with the skin or various mucous membranes of the organs or through the bloodstream after absorption. Almost any part of the body can be affected by allergies.

Allergic reactions are caused by a wide range of substances and conditions. These include pollens, dust, cosmetics, and animal hair; poisonous plants, serums, vaccines, and drugs; physical agents such as heat, cold and sunlight, as well as a variety of foods. The foods that commonly cause allergic reactions are oranges, milk,

---

1. For further information, see chapters on Asthma and Eczema

eggs, wheat, fish and other sea foods, chocolates, tomatoes, and strawberries.

Causes and Symptoms

Allergic symptoms are manifested in various forms in different organs. These include recurring headaches, migraines, dizziness, irritability. nervousness, depression, neuralgia, conjunctivitis, eczema, hay fever, a stuffy or runny nose, diarrhoea, vomiting, urticaria, asthma, shortness of breath, and swelling of the face and eyes. The same substance can cause different symptoms in different people at different times.

Allergy is an indication of disharmony caused by dietetic errors and a faulty style of living. It is also caused by excessive consumption of refined and processed foods, loaded with numerous chemical additives, many of which cause powerful reactions. Emotional and psychological stress can also lead to allergies.

Remedies

Nutrients: Certain nutrients have been found beneficial in the prevention and treatment of allergies. Often the intake of vitamin B$_5$ or pantothenic acid brings great relief to the sufferer. This vitamin may be taken in a dose of 100 mg daily for a month. In such cases, liberal amounts of pantothenic acid helps even though the recovery takes several weeks. A dose of 400 mg of vitamin E taken daily for four to six weeks is also beneficial as this vitamin possesses effective anti-allergic properties.

Castor Oil: An effective home remedy for allergy has been discovered by an Indian physician, Dr Hemant Pathak. He found that five drops of castor oil in half a cup of any fruit or vegetable juice, or plain water, and taken on an empty stomach in the morning, is beneficial for allergies of the intestinal tract, skin, and nasal passages. Dr Pathak has reported numerous cases of allergic protection by this method.[1]

Lime: Lime is considered an effective remedy for any kind of allergy. Half a lime may be squeezed in a glass of lukewarm water and sweetened with a teaspoon of honey. It can be taken once daily first thing in the morning for several months. This remedy not only flushes the system of toxins but also acts as an antitoxic and antiallergic agent. However, those who are allergic to citrus fruits should not take recourse to this remedy.

---

1. Linda Clark, *A Handbook for Natural Remedies for Common Ailments,* First Edition, p. 32, Pocket Books, New York, 1977.

Bananas: One or two bananas a day are useful for those who are allergic to certain foods and who consequently suffer from skin rashes, digestive disorders, or asthma. The fruit does, however, cause allergic reactions in certain sensitive persons and they should avoid it.

Vegetable Juices: A quantity of 500 ml carrot juice or a combination of carrot juice with beet and cucumber juices, has been found beneficial in the treatment of allergies. In the case of mixed juices, 100 ml each of beet and cucumber juices should be mixed with 300 ml of carrot juice to prepare 500 ml or half a litre of mixed juice. This should be taken once daily.

Dietary Considerations

The best way to prevent or overcome allergies is to strengthen overall physical resistance so as not to fall an easy prey to every allergen that one comes across. To start with, the patient should fast on fresh fruit juices for four or five days. Repeated short juice fasts are likely to result in better tolerance to previous allergies. After the juice fast, the patient can take a mono diet of vegetables or fruits such as carrots, grapes, or apples for one week. After that, one more food may be added to the mono diet. A week later, a third food may be added, and so on. After four weeks, protein foods can be introduced, one at a time. In case an allergic reaction to a newly-introduced food is noticed, it should be discontinued and a new food tried. In this way, all real allergens can be eventually eliminated from the diet.

Foods which should be excluded from the diet are tea, coffee, chocolate, cola drinks, alcohol, sugar and products made from it, refined cereals, meats, fish, chicken, tobacco, milk, cheese, butter, smoked and salted pickled foods, and foods containing any chemical additives, preservatives and flavourings.

Other Measures

For allergic conditions in which an element of mental stress is present as well, it is essential to employ such methods as relaxation, exercise, meditation, and mind control. These methods reduce or remove stress and thereby contribute towards the treatment of allergies. Yogic *asanas* like *yogamudra, ardh-matsyendrasana, sarvangasana, shavasana,* and *anuloma-viloma pranayama* are beneficial in the treatment of allergy.

Amnesia

Amnesia refers to partial or complete loss of memory. Different types and degrees of amnesia occur in old age and in some mental disorders.

Causes and Symptoms

The most common form of this disease is verbal amnesia. In this condition, the patient forgets words or names. An uncommon form of amnesia is temporary loss of memory, in which a person even forgets his own identity, including his name, age, family background, and any recollection of the past.

The main cause of amnesia is the impairment of brain cells by diseases which affect them directly or indirectly, due to a poor blood supply caused by circulatory diseases. Poor memory also results from dullness of intellect and weakness of the brain. Many cases are, however, largely psychological in origin. They are caused by anxiety neurosis, resulting from attention-seeking in persons obsessed with their own problems. Temporary loss of memory may result from an injury.

Remedies

Rosemary: The most remarkable remedy for loss of memory or forgetfulness is the use of the herb rosemary, botanically known as *Romarinus officinalis*. Rosemary has long been regarded as a herb for remembrance. In ancient times, the Greeks and the Romans prepared fragrant distilled water from the flowers of this plant and inhaled the odour so that 'the evils were destroyed from the mind and the memory no longer played tricks.'[1] Rosemary is considered to be an antidote for mental fatigue and forgetfulness. A tea made from this herb, taken once or twice a day, is a refreshing drink and an effective natural remedy for enhancing mental agility.

Brahmi Booti: Another herb useful in amnesia is *brahmi booti*, botanically known as *Bacopa scrophulariaceae*. About seven grams of this herb should be dried in the shade and ground in water, along with seven kernels of almonds and half a gram of pepper.

---

1. Lucas Richard, *The Magic of Herbs in Daily Living*, Parker Publishing House, New York, 1972.

16

This mixture should be strained and sweetened with twenty-five gm of sugar. It should be drunk every morning for a fortnight on an empty stomach.

Sage: The herb sage has also been found beneficial in the treatment of a weak memory or loss of memory. It acts on the cortex of the brain, mitigates mental exhaustion and strengthens the ability to concentrate. A tea prepared from dried sage leaves can be used regularly for this purpose.

Almonds: Almonds are very valuable for restoring a poor memory caused by brain weakness. They contain unique properties to remove brain debility and to strengthen the brain. Almonds preserve the vitality of the brain and cure ailments originating from nervous disorders. Ten to twelve almonds should be immersed in water overnight and their outer skin removed. They should then be made into a fine paste and taken, mixed with one teaspoonful of butter or even alone. Inhaling ten to fifteen drops of almond oil through the nose, morning and evening, is also beneficial in the treatment of brain weakness.

Walnuts: Walnut is another unique dry fruit valuable in countering brain weakness. About twenty grams of walnuts should be taken every day. The value of walnuts is enhanced if they are taken with figs or raisins in a proportion of ten gram each, everyday.

Apples: Apples are useful in amnesia. The various chemical substances contained in this fruit such as vitamin B_1, phosphorus, and potassium help in the synthesis of glutamic acid. This acid controls the wear and tear of nerve cells. Eating an apple a day with one tea-spoon of honey and one cup of milk is beneficial in the treatment of loss of memory and mental irritability. It acts as an effective nerve tonic and recharges the nerves with new energy and life.

Other Fruits: All fruits which are rich in phosphorus are valuable mitigators of amnesia, as they invigorate the brain cells and tissues. Apart from apples, almonds, and walnuts, which have been discussed earlier, other phosphorus-rich fruits are figs, grapes, oranges, and dates. Their intake is highly beneficial in loss of memory due to brain debility.

Cumin Seeds: The use of cumin seeds is another valuable remedy for amnesia or dullness of memory. Three grams of black cumin seeds should be mixed with two teaspoonfuls of pure honey and taken once a day, preferably, in the morning.

Black Pepper: Five seeds of finely ground black pepper, mixed with one teaspoon of honey are also beneficial in the treatment of this condition. This preparation should be taken both in the morning and evening.

Dietary Considerations

The diet of a patient suffering from amnesia should consist of phosphorus-rich foods like cereals, pulses, nuts, egg yolk, fruit juices, and milk. Cow's milk is specially beneficial and the patient should take as much of this milk as he can safely digest.

Other Measures

Ensuring sufficient rest and sleep under conducive conditions is very necessary. The patient must also learn the art of relaxation and meditation which can go a long way in curing amnesia.

Anaemia

Haemoglobin Deficiency in Blood

Anaemia may be defined as a condition in which there is a decrease in the quantity of haemoglobin or in the number of red cells. Anaemia is among the most common ailments affecting human beings.

Nearly half the blood flowing in our veins and arteries consists of red blood cells which carry oxygen to the tissues. Approximately one trillion or 100 million new blood cells are formed daily in the bone marrow. The raw materials required in the production of these cells are iron, proteins, and vitamins, especially folic acid and B_{12}. Of these, iron and proteins are essential in building up the red colouring matter called haemoglobin. A red cell has a lifespan of approximately one hundred and twenty days and is then destroyed and replaced. Each person should have about 15 gm of haemoglobin per 100 ml of blood, and a blood count of approximately five million red cells per millimetre of blood.

Causes and Symptoms

The patient usually complains of weakness, fatigue, lack of energy, and dizziness. Other symptoms include a haggard look, premature wrinkles, dull and tired looking eyes, poor memory, shortness of breath on exertion, headache, slow healing of wounds, and palpitations. The skin and mucous membranes look pale.

A diminished formation of red blood cells in the bone marrow, either due to defects in the bone marrow, or due to an inadequate intake of iron, vitamins, and proteins, is one of the main causes of anaemia. Other important causes are heavy loss of blood due to injury, bleeding piles, or excessive menstruation in women. Anaemia can also occur due to a lack of hydrochloric acid in the stomach, which is needed for digestion of iron and proteins, or intestinal parasites or worms. Hookworms, pinworms, round worms and tape worms feed on the supply of blood as well as on the vitamins.

Remedies

Vitamin B$_{12}$: Vitamin B$_{12}$ is needed for preventing or curing anaemia. This vitamin is usually found in animal protein, especially in meats such as kidney and liver. There are, however, other equally good sources of vitamin B$_{12}$ such as dairy products which also contain some B$_{12}$.

Beets: Beets are very helpful in curing anaemia. Beet juice contains potassium, phosphorus, calcium, sulphur, iodine, iron, copper, carbohydrates, protein, fat, vitamins B$_1$, B$_2$, B$_6$, niacin, and vitamin P. With their high iron content, beets help in the formation of red blood cells. The juice of red beet strengthens the body's powers of resistance and has proved to be an excellent remedy for anaemia, especially for children and teenagers, where other blood-forming remedies have failed.

Fenugreek: The leaves of fenugreek help in blood formation. The cooked leaves should be taken by adolescent girls to prevent anaemia, which may occur due to the onset of puberty and menstruation. The seeds of fenugreek are also a valuable cure for anaemia, being rich in iron.

Lettuce: Lettuce is another effective remedy for this ailment as it contains a considerable amount of iron. It can, therefore, be used as a good tonic food for anaemia. The iron in it is easily absorbed by the body.

Spinach: This leafy vegetable is a valuable source of high grade iron. After its absorption, it helps in the formation of haemoglobin and red blood cells. It is thus beneficial in building up the blood, and in the prevention and treatment of anaemia.

Soyabean: Soyabean is rich in iron and also has a high protein value. As most anaemic patients usually also suffer from a weak digestion, it should be given to them in a very light form, preferably in the form of milk, which can be easily digested.

Almonds: Almonds contain copper to the extent of 1.15 mg per 100 gm. The copper along with iron and vitamins, acts as a catalyst in the synthesis of haemoglobin. Almonds are, therefore, a useful remedy for anaemia. Seven almonds should be soaked in water for about two hours and ground into a paste after removing the thin red skin. This paste may be eaten once daily in the morning for three months.

Sesame Seeds: Black sesame seeds, as a rich source of iron, are valuable in anaemia. After soaking one teaspoon of the seeds in warm water for a couple of hours, they should be ground and strained, and then mixed with a cup of milk and sweetened with jaggery or sugar. This emulsion should be given to patients suffering from anaemia.

Honey: Honey is remarkable for building haemoglobin in the body. This is largely due to the iron, copper, and manganese contained in it.

Other Foods: There are several other foods which are rich sources of iron and can be used beneficially in the treatment of anaemia. The more important of these are bananas, black grapes, plums, strawberries, raisins, onions, squash, carrots, radish, celery, and tomatoes.

Dietary Considerations

Diet is of utmost importance in the treatment of anaemia. Refined foods like white bread, polished rice, sugar, and desserts rob the body of its much-needed iron. Iron should preferably be taken in its natural organic form in food. The emphasis in the diet should be on raw vegetables and fresh fruits which are rich in iron.

The patient should commence a therapeutic treatment with an exclusive fruit diet for five days, taking three meals a day of fresh juicy fruits. This may be followed by a fruit and milk diet for about fifteen days. In this regimen, the frequency of meals should be exactly the same as for the earlier all-fruit diet. Thereafter, the patient may gradually embark upon a well-balanced diet, consisting of seeds, nuts, grains, vegetables, and fruits.

Other Measures

Cold water baths are recommended in anaemia. The patient

should be given a cold bath carefully twice daily, the coldness of the water being increased gradually. A hot Epsom salts bath for five to ten minutes once a week and an occasional steam bath are also useful. Sunbaths are especially beneficial as the sunlight stimulates the production of red cells. Other important factors that help in curing anaemia are deep breathing and light exercises like walking. Yogic *asanas* such as *sarvangasana, paschimottanasana,* and *shavasana,* as well as massage are also helpful in this regard.

Anorexia

Loss of Appetite

Anorexia means loss of appetite. It is a symptom of disturbed digestion and common in all diseases which lead to general weakness. This condition results from failure of the activity of the stomach and secretion of gastric juices due to low vitality which, in turn, can be due to various causes.

Causes and Symptoms

Persons suffering from anorexia may refuse to eat and suffer from insomnia. In course of time, emaciation becomes severe.

People suffer from anorexia when they habitually take a faulty diet and hardly do any physical work. It may also result from stress and strain such as domestic worry, emotional disturbances, difficult working conditions, and nervous disorders. General body disorders and diseases also lead to this condition.

Remedies

Oranges: Oranges are an extremely useful remedy for anorexia. They stimulate the flow of digestive juices, thereby improving digestion and increasing appetite. One or two oranges a day are advised.

Sour Grapes: Sour grapes are another effective remedy for anorexia. The juice of these grapes should be used in kneading the flour before preparing *chapatis. Chapatis* made in this manner should be eaten continuously for two to three weeks. This remedy will tone up the stomach and improve the appetite.

21

Lime: Lime is also a valuable remedy for restoring a lost appetite. A preparation made from this fruit and ginger has been found very effective in overcoming this condition. About one teaspoon of the juice of lime should be mixed with an equal quantity of the juice of ginger. One gram of rock salt should be added to this mixture. It should then be placed in sunlight for three days. A teaspoon taken after each meal will tone up the digestive system and improve the appetite.

Apples: Apples are another variety of fruit useful in anorexia. They help digestion by stimulating the flow of pepsin, a protein-digesting enzyme, in the stomach. The old adage, 'An apple a day keeps the doctor away', is certainly a valuable one.

Garlic: Garlic possesses a special property to stimulate the digestive tone of the system and improve appetite. A soup prepared from this vegetable can be of immense help to a patient suffering from anorexia. Three or four cloves of raw garlic should be boiled in a cup of water. This soup can be reinforced with the juice of half a lemon and taken twice daily.

Ginger: The use of ginger is valuable in the loss of appetite. About five grams of this vegetable should be ground and licked with a little salt once a day for the treatment of this condition.

Dietary Considerations

The only effective treatment for anorexia is a thorough cleansing of the digestive tract, and adoption of a sensible diet thereafter, along with a change in the style of living. To begin with, the patient should fast on orange juice and water for three to five days. The procedure is to take the juice of an orange in a glass of warm water, every two hours, from 8 a.m. to 8 p.m. Nothing else should be taken, as otherwise, the value of the fast will be entirely lost. If orange juice does not agree with the system, only water or half a glass of carrot juice mixed with an equal quantity of water may be taken. After the juice fast, the patient may adopt an all-fruit diet for a further five days, taking three meals a day of juicy fruits, such as apples, pears, grapes, grape-fruit, oranges, pineapple, peaches, and melons, at five-hourly intervals. Thereafter he may adopt a restricted diet of easily-digestible foods, consisting of lightly cooked vegetables, juicy fruits, and butter milk for about ten days.

Other Measures

During the first three to five days of the juice fast, the bowels should be cleansed with a warm-water enema each day. The poisonous matter will thus be eliminated by this self-cleansing process.

The application of an ice-bag over the stomach for half an hour before meals, and a cool hip bath once or twice daily, will go a long way in curing anorexia. Other measures beneficial in the treatment of this condition are sun and cool air baths. An early morning sun bath, taken one day, should be alternated with an early morning cool air bath the next day. An outdoor life and abdominal massages are also advised.

Appendicitis

Inflammation of Appendix

The appendix is a small outgrowth of tissue forming a tube-shaped sac attached to the lower end of the large intestine. Inflammation of the appendix presents itself in acute and chronic forms and affects both the sexes equally. This disease accounts for about half the acute abdominal emergencies occurring between the ages of ten and thirty.

Causes and Symptoms

Appendicitis usually begins with a sudden pain in the centre of the abdomen. The pain may be preceded by general discomfort in the abdomen, indigestion, diarrhoea, or constipation. Gradually, the pain shifts to the lower right side, and is usually accompanied by a fever varying from 38^0C to 39^0C. Nausea is common and the patient may vomit once or twice. In the chronic state of appendicitis, the patient may suffer from recurrent pain in the right lower abdomen, constipation, loss of appetite, and mild nausea.

Appendicitis is initiated by the presence of an excessive amount of poisonous waste material in the caecum. As a result, the appendix gets irritated and inflamed. Inflammation and infection are caused by certain germs which are usually present in the intestinal tract.

Remedies

When pains as described above are experienced, the patient is advised to consult a doctor immediately. The following remedies should be taken only in consultation with a doctor:

Green Gram: Green gram is a proven home remedy for acute appendicitis. An infusion of green gram is an excellent medicine for treating this condition. It can be taken in a small quantity of one tablespoon three times a day.

Fenugreek Seeds: Regular use of tea made from fenugreek seeds has proved helpful in preventing the appendix from becoming a dumping ground for excess mucus and intestinal waste. This tea is prepared by putting one tablespoon of the seeds in a litre of cold water and allowing it to simmer for half an hour over a low flame and then strained it. It should be allowed to cool a little before being drunk.

Vegetable Juices: Certain vegetable juices have been found valuable in appendicitis. A particularly good combination is that of 100 ml each of beet and cucumber juices mixed with 300 ml of carrot juice. This combined juice can be taken twice daily.

Buttermilk: Buttermilk is beneficial in the treatment of chronic form of appendicitis. One litre of buttermilk may be taken daily for this purpose.

Whole Wheat: The consumption of whole wheat, which includes bran and wheat germ, has been found beneficial in preventing several digestive disorders, including appendicitis. The bran of wheat can be sterilised by baking after thorough cleaning. This sterilised bran can be added to wheat flour in the proportion of one to six by weight. Two or three *chapatis* made from this flour can be eaten daily for preventing this disease.

Dietary Considerations

At the first symptoms of severe pain, vomiting, and fever, the patient should resort to fasting and nothing except water should enter the system. Fruit juices may be given from the third day onwards for the next three days. Thereafter the patient may adopt an all-fruit diet for a further four or five days. After this tightly regulated regimen, he should adopt a well-balanced diet, consisting of seeds, nuts, grains, vegetables, and fruits.

Other Measures

When the first symptoms of pain, vomiting, and fever occur, the patient must be put to bed immediately, as rest is of the utmost importance. A low enema, containing about half a litre of warm water, should be administered once every day for the first three days to cleanse the lower bowel if it can be tolerated with comfort.

Hot compresses may be placed over the painful area several times daily. Abdominal packs, made of a strip of wet sheet and covered by a dry flannel cloth bound tightly around the abdomen, should be applied continuously until all acute symptoms subside.

When the acute symptoms subside by about the third day, the patient should be given a full enema, containing about three litres of warm water, and this should be repeated daily until all inflammation and pain have subsided.

In other words, the patient of appendicitis should adopt all measures to eradicate constipation. Once the waste matter in the caecum has moved into the colon and is then eliminated, the irritation and inflammation in the appendix will subside and surgical removal of the appendix may not be necessary.

Arteriosclerosis

Narrowing of the Arteries

Arteriosclerosis refers to the thickening of the walls of the arteries. It has become a common ailment in modern times, accounting for much of the disability and high death rate, more so among older people.

Arteriosclerosis is usually preceded by atherosclerosis, a kind of fatty infiltration in the inner lining of the blood vessel walls. The most risky places for such degeneration are the coronary vessels of the heart and the arteries of the brain. Arteriosclerosis results in the loss of elasticity of the blood vessels and a narrowing of the smaller arteries, which interferes with the free circulation of the blood.

Causes and Symptoms

The symptoms of arteriosclerosis vary according to the arteries involved. Signs of inadequate blood supply generally appear first in the legs. There may be numbness and coldness in the feet, and cramps and pains in the legs even after light exercise. If the coronary arteries are involved, the patient may have sharp pains, characteristic of angina pectoris. When arteries leading to the brain are involved, the vessel may burst, causing haemorrhage in the brain tissues. A cerebral vascular stroke, with partial or complete paralysis on one side of the body, may result if there is blockage with a blood clot. It may also lead to loss of memory and a confused state of mind in elderly people. If arteries leading to the kidneys are involved, the patient may suffer from high blood pressure and kidney disorders.

The most important causes of arteriosclerosis are lack of physical exercise, excessive intake of white sugar, refined foods, and a high fat diet rich in cholesterol. Hardening of the arteries may also be caused by other diseases such as high blood pressure, obesity, and diabetes. Emotional stress plays an important part, and heart attacks are more common during periods of mental and emotional disturbances, particularly in those engaged in sedentary occupations. Heredity also plays its role and this disease runs in families.

Remedies

It is imperative that a patient has his condition diagnosed by a physician and resorts to remedies only in consultation with him.

Lemon: One of the most effective home remedies for arteriosclerosis is the lemon peel. It is believed to be one of the richest sources of vitamin P. It strengthens the entire arterial system. Shredded lemon peel of one lemon may be added to soups and stews, or sprinkled over salads. To make a medicine, the peel of one or two lemons may be cut up finely, covered with warm water and allowed to stand for about twelve hours. A teaspoon may be taken every three hours, or immediately before or after a meal.

Parsley: Parsley is another effective remedy for arteriosclerosis. It contains elements which help to maintain the blood vessels, particularly the capillaries, and arterial system in a healthy condition. It may be taken as a tea: a teaspoon of dry parsley may be allowed to simmer gently in a cupful of water for a few minutes. This can be taken two to three times daily.

Vegetable Juices: Beet juice, taken daily, has been found valuable in arteriosclerosis. It is an excellent solvent for inorganic calcium deposits. The juices of carrots and spinach are also beneficial if taken once a day. These juices can be taken individually—500 ml, or as a combination. When taken as a combination, they should be in the following proportion: carrots—300 ml and spinach—200 ml to prepare 500 ml of juice.

Honey: Honey is also considered beneficial in the treatment of arteriosclerosis. It is easily digested and assimilated. The patient should take a glass of water with one teaspoon each of honey and lemon juice in it, before going to bed. He can also take it if he wakes up at night.

Ishabgul: The herb ishabgul, botanically known as *Plantago-ovata*, has been found valuable in arteriosclerosis. The oil of the seeds of this plant should be used. It contains fifty per cent of linoleic acid, an unsaturated fat, and is, therefore, helpful in the prevention and treatment of this disease.

Garlic and Onions: Recent investigations have shown that garlic and onions have a preventive effect on the development of arteriosclerosis. They should be included in the daily diet, either raw or cooked, according to individual taste.

Dietary Considerations

To begin with, the patient should resort to a juice fast for five to seven days. Fresh, raw vegetables and juices of seasonal fruits may be taken three times a day. After the juice fast, the patient should take a diet consisting of seeds, nuts, grains, vegetables, and fruits, with emphasis on raw foods. Further short fasts of juices may be undertaken at intervals of three months or so, depending on the progress being made.

The patient should take several small meals instead of a few large ones. He should avoid all hydrogenated fats and an excess of saturated fats, such as butter, cream, ghee, and animal fat. Vegetable oils, particularly safflower oil, flax seed oil, and olive oil, should be used as a cooking medium. He should also avoid meat, salt, and all refined and processed foods, condiments, sauces, pickles, strong tea, coffee, white sugar, white flour, and all products made from them.

Other Measures

During the juice fast undertaken for the first five to seven days, a warm-water enema should be used daily to cleanse the bowels.

Smoking, if habitual, should be given up as it constricts the arteries and aggravates the condition. The patient should undertake plenty of outdoor exercise and learn to take mental stress and worries in his stride. A prolonged immersion bath at room temperature should be taken at bedtime on alternate days. This bath should be administered in a bath tub properly fitted with a hot and cold water connection. The bath tub should be filled with water at a temperature ranging from 33.4^0C to 36.7^0C, and the

27

patient should lie in it for an hour or so. The head should be kept cold with a cold compress.

Arthritis

The word 'arthritis' means 'inflammation of the joints'. It is derived from two Greek words: *athron,* meaning joints; and *itis,* meaning inflammation. It is, generally, a chronic disease process.

Arthritis occurs in various forms, the most frequent being osteoarthritis and rheumatoid arthritis. Osteoarthritis is a degenerative joint disease which usually occurs in the older age-group. Rheumatoid arthritis is a serious disease which affects not only the joints of the fingers, wrists, hips, knees, and feet, but also the muscles, tendons and other tissues of the body.

Causes and Symptoms

The main symptoms of osteoarthritis are pain and stiffness in the joints. The pain usually increases after exercise. Rheumatoid arthritis is often called the 'cooked food disease'. It usually develops gradually over several months, with persistent pain and stiffness in one or more joints. Ultimately the whole body is affected. Symptoms include anaemia, colitis, constipation, deformed hands and feet.

Osteoarthritis results from structural changes in the articular cartilage in the joints, usually those which are weight-bearing, such as the spine and knees. Rheumatoid arthritis is due to an inflammation of the synovium or lining of the joints. This is accompanied by swelling and eventually leads to deformity. The condition may be caused by hormonal imbalance, physical and emotional stress, infection, severe fright, shock, and injury. Hereditary factors may also be responsible for the onset of this disease.

Remedies

Potato Juice: The raw potato juice therapy is considered one of the most successful biological treatments for rheumatic and arthritic conditions. It has been used in folk medicine for centuries. The traditional method of preparing potato juice is to cut a medium-sized potato into thin slices, without peeling the skin, and place the slices overnight in a large glass filled with cold water. The water should be drunk in the morning on an empty stomach. Fresh juice can also be extracted from potatoes. A medium-sized potato should be diluted with a cup of water and drunk first thing in the morning.

Other Raw Juices: One cup of green juice, extracted from any green leafy vegetable, mixed in equal proportions with carrot, celery, and red beet juices is good for arthritis. The alkaline action of raw juices dissolves the accumulation of deposits around the joints and in other tissues. A cup of fresh pineapple juice is also valuable, as the enzyme bromelain in fresh pineapple juice reduces swelling and inflammation in osteoarthritis and rheumatoid arthritis.

Sesame Seeds: A teaspoon of black sesame seeds, soaked in a quarter cup of water and kept overnight, has been found to be effective in preventing frequent joint pains. The water in which the seeds are soaked should also be taken along with the seeds first thing in the morning.

Copper: Drinking water kept overnight in a copper container accumulates traces of copper, which is said to strengthen the muscular system. A copper ring or bracelet is worn for the same reason.

Calcium: Studies have shown that calcium can help arthritis.[1] Several patients have discovered that joint pains have either been relieved or have disappeared entirely after taking calcium. This mineral should be taken in the form of calcium lactate. Two teaspoons of calcium lactate, each teaspoon providing 400 mg of absorbable calcium, may be taken three times daily in water, before meals for at least four months.

Garlic: Garlic is another effective remedy for arthritis. It contains an anti-inflammatory property which accounts for its effectiveness in the treatment of this disease. Garlic may be taken raw or cooked according to individual preference.

Bananas: Bananas, being a rich source of vitamin B_6, have proved useful in the treatment of arthritis. A diet of only bananas for three or four days is advised in treating this condition. The patient may eat eight or nine bananas daily during this period and nothing else.

Lime: Lime has also been found beneficial as a home remedy for arthritis. The citric acid found in lime is a solvent of uric acid which is the primary cause of some types of arthritis. The juice

1. Mark Bricklin, *Natural Home Remedies*, Rodale Press, 1986.

29

of one lime, diluted with water, may be taken once a day, preferably first thing in the morning.

Alfalfa: A tea made from the herb alfalfa, especially from its seeds, has shown beneficial results in the treatment of arthritis. One teaspoon of alfalfa seeds may be added to one cup of water. Three to four cups of this tea should be taken daily by arthritics for at least two weeks.

Green Gram Soup: Another home remedy found useful in relieving pains in the joints is the use of green gram soup. This soup should be prepared by mixing a tablespoon of green gram in a cup of water, with two crushed garlic cloves. It should be taken twice a day.

Castor Oil: Treatment with castor oil has been found beneficial in arthritis. The procedure, as prescribed by a Spanish doctor, is to boil two tablespoons of castor oil over a stove burner. The oil should then be poured into a glass of fresh orange juice and taken before breakfast daily till the disease is cured. This treatment is believed to have been adopted by an American doctor, called Dr Taylor, in 1900. He advised his patients to take it for three weeks, wait for another three weeks and then repeat it again for another three weeks. It is, however, essential that the patient must take an alkaline diet while adopting this mode of treatment; otherwise the value of the treatment will be lost.[2]

Coconut or Mustard Oil: Warm coconut oil or mustard oil, mixed with two or three pieces of camphor should be massaged on stiff and aching joints. It will increase blood supply, and reduce inflammation and stiffness with the gentle warmth produced while massaging. Camphorated oil is an ancient rubefacient used for the purpose.

Dietary Considerations

The diet of an arthritis patient should be planned so as to produce alkalinity in the blood. It should include fruits and vegetables in the form of salads, and, at least, two cooked vegetables. In severe cases, it would be advisable to put the patient on raw vegetable juice therapy three times a day, for about a week. Repeated juice fasts are recommended at intervals of every two months.

---

2. Article titled 'Herbal Treatment for Arthritis' by Joe A. Lewis in *Body and Beauty Care* magazine, Bombay, June 30, 1992 issue.

Other Measures

The body should be kept warm at all times. Joints should not be bandaged tightly as this limits movement and interferes with the free circulation of blood. There should be plenty of indirect ventilation in the bedroom. Rest is advised when there is acute inflammation in the joints.

Sea bathing has been found valuable in arthritis. The natural iodine in sea water is said to relieve arthritis pain. As is well known, iodine regulates the acid-alkaline balance in the blood and tissues, helps to repair and regenerate worn out tissues and nourishes the skeletal structure. It enters into the thyroid gland's secretion. The hormone uses the iodine to cleanse the internal toxins.

If sea bathing is not possible, the patient should relax for thirty minutes every night in a tub of warm water, in which a cup of common salt has been mixed. The minerals in the salt, especially iodine, will be absorbed through the pores of the skin. This will help correct an internal imbalance.

Asthma

Bronchial Asthma

Asthma is an ancient Greek word meaning 'panting or short-drawn breath'. It is an allergic condition resulting from the reaction of the body to one or more allergens, and is the most troublesome of respiratory diseases. An asthma patient gets frequent attacks of breathlessness, in between which he may even be completely normal.

Causes and Symptoms

Patients suffering from asthma appear to be gasping for breath. Actually, they have more difficulty in breathing out than breathing in, and this is caused by spasms or sudden involuntary muscular contractions of the smaller air passages in the lungs. The effect is to blow the lungs up because the patient cannot drive the air properly out of the lungs before he has to take another breath. Most asthmatics have more difficulty at night or early morning.

Asthma is caused by a variety of factors. It may be due to an allergy caused by weather conditions, food, drugs, perfumes, and other irritants. Allergies to dust are the most common. Foods which generally cause allergic reactions are wheat, eggs, milk, chocolates, beans, fish, and sea foods. The disease may also result from psychological factors. According to some studies, about twenty-five per cent of young asthmatics have a deep-seated emotional insecurity and an intense need for parental love and protection. Heredity also plays an important role.

Remedies

Honey: Honey is one of the most common home remedies for asthma. It is said that if a jug of honey is held under the nose of an asthma patient and he inhales the air that comes into contact with it, he starts breathing easier and deeper. The effect lasts for an hour or so. One to two teaspoonfuls of honey provide relief. Honey can also be taken in a cup of milk or water. Honey thins out accumulated mucus and helps its elimination from the respiratory passages. It also tones up the pulmonary lining and thereby prevents the production of mucus in future. Some authorities recommend one-year old honey for asthma and respiratory diseases.[1]

Figs: Among fruits, figs have proved very valuable in asthma. They give comfort to the patient by draining off the phlegm. Three or four dry figs should be cleaned thoroughly with warm water and soaked overnight. They should be taken first thing in the morning, along with the water in which they were soaked. This treatment may be continued for about two months.

Lemon: Lemon is another fruit found beneficial in the treatment of asthma. The juice of one lemon, diluted in a glass of water and taken with meals, will bring good results.

Indian Gooseberry: Indian gooseberry has also proved valuable in asthma. Five grams of gooseberry mixed with one tablespoon of honey forms an effective medicinal tonic for the treatment of this disease. It should be taken every morning. When fresh fruit is not available, dry gooseberry powder can be mixed with honey.

Bitter Gourd Roots: The roots of the bitter gourd plant have been used in folk medicine for asthma since ancient times.

---

1. P.E. Norris, *About Honey,* 4th Edition, Thorsons Publishers Ltd., Great Britain, 1981.

A teaspoon of the root paste, mixed with an equal amount of honey or juice of the *tulsi* leaves, given once every night for a month, acts as an excellent medicine for this disease.

Drumstick Leaves: A soup prepared from drumstick leaves, and taken once daily, has been found beneficial in the treatment of asthma. This soup is prepared by adding a handful of leaves to 180 ml of water and boiling it for five minutes. After being allowed to cool, a little salt, pepper, and lime juice may be added to this soup.

Ginger: A teaspoon of fresh ginger juice, mixed with a cup of fenugreek decoction and honey to taste, acts as an excellent expectorant in cases of asthma. The decoction of fenugreek can be made by mixing one tablespoon of fenugreek seeds in a cupful of water. This remedy should be taken once in the morning and once in the evening.

Garlic: Garlic is another effective home remedy for asthma. Ten garlic cloves, boiled in 30 ml of milk, make an excellent medicine for the early stages of asthma. This mixture should be taken once daily by the patient. Steaming ginger tea with two minced garlic cloves in it, can also help to keep the problem under control, and should be taken in the morning and evening.

Bishop's Weed: The herb bishop's weed has been found valuable in asthma. Half a teaspoon of bishop's weed should be mixed in a glass of buttermilk and taken twice daily. It is an effective remedy for relieving difficult expectoration caused by dried-up phlegm. A hot poultice of the seeds should be used for dry fomentation to the chest, twice daily. The patient can also inhale steam twice a day from boiling water mixed with *ajwain*. It will dilate the bronchial passages.

Safflower: Safflower seeds are beneficial in the treatment of bronchial asthma. Half a teaspoon of powder of the dry seeds, mixed with a tablespoon of honey, can be taken once or twice a day in treating this disease. This acts as an expectorant and reduces the spasms by liquefying the tenacious sputum. An infusion of five grams of flowers mixed with one tablespoon of honey, taken once daily, is also useful in this disease.

Linseed: A decoction of linseed is also considered useful in curing congestion in asthma and preventing recurrence of attacks. The decoction is prepared by boiling a teaspoon of linseed powder and a piece of palm candy in two cups of water till the mixture is reduced to half. This decoction taken with a tablespoon of milk once daily, will provide relief from chest congestion. Simultaneously, a linseed poultice should be applied externally during the attack, at the lung bases.

Mustard Oil: During the attack, mustard oil, mixed with a little camphor, should be massaged over the back of the chest. This will loosen up phlegm and ease breathing

Copper: One of the preventive measures to stop attacks of asthma is to drink water which has been kept overnight in a copper vessel. This water, with traces of copper in it, is believed to change one's constitutional tendency to get respiratory problems.

Dietary Considerations

The patient should avoid common dietetic errors. Ideally, his diet should contain a limited quantity of carbohydrates, fats, and proteins which are 'acid-forming' foods, and a liberal quantity of alkali-forming foods consisting of fresh fruits, green vegetables, sprouted seeds, and grains. The patient should avoid foods which tend to produce phlegm, such as rice, sugar, lentils, and curds. He should also avoid fried and other difficult-to-digest foods, strong tea, coffee, alcoholic beverages, condiments, pickles, sauces, and all refined and processed foods.

Other Measures

The patient should also follow the other laws of nature. Air, sun, and water are great healing agents. Regular fasting once a week, an occasional enema, breathing exercises, fresh air, a dry climate, light exercises, and correct posture go a long way in treating the disease.

Backache

Spondylosis, Lumbago

Backache is one of the most common ailments prevalent today. Sedentary living habits, hazardous work patterns and psychological conditions associated with emotional stress, which bring about spasm of the muscles, cause backaches. As the back bears the weight of the entire body, overweight persons feel the strain on the back when they have to carry an extra load.

Causes and Symptoms

In most cases of backache, the pain is usually felt either in the middle of the back or lower down. It may spread to both sides of the waist and the hips. In a condition of acute pain, the patient is unable to move and is bedridden.

About ninety per cent of backache patients suffer from what is called cervical and lumbar spondylosis. It is a degenerative disorder in which the different vertebrae adhere to each other through bony unions. As a result of this, the spine loses its flexibility.

The main causes of backache and spondylosis are muscular tension, straining of the joints, poor posture, and incorrect nutrition resulting from dietetic errors and lack of exercise. Acute or chronic illnesses like kidney or prostate problems, female disorders, influenza, and arthritis, may also lead to backache. Other causes include stress and strain resulting from sitting for a long time, improper lifting of weights, high heels, and emotional problems which may cause painful muscle cramping.

Remedies

Garlic: The most important home remedy for backache is the use of garlic. Two or three cloves should be taken every morning to get results. An oil prepared from garlic and rubbed on the back will give great relief. This oil is prepared by frying ten cloves of garlic in 60 ml of oil in a frying pan. Any of the oils which are used as rubefacients, such as mustard oil, sesame oil, and coconut oil can be used according to one's choice. They should be fried on a slow fire till they are brown. After the oil has cooled, it should be applied vigorously on the back, and allowed to remain there for three hours. The patient may, thereafter, take a warm-water bath. This treatment should be continued for at least fifteen days.

Lemon: Lemon is another useful remedy for backache. The juice of one lemon should be mixed with common salt and taken by the patient twice daily. It will give relief.

Chebulic Myroblan: The use of chebulic myroblan is beneficial in the treatment of backache. A small piece of this fruit should be eaten after meals. This will give quick relief.

Vitamin C: Vitamin C has proved valuable in case of severe backaches. About 2,000 mg of this vitamin should be taken daily for treating this condition. Considerable improvement will be noticeable within two days.

Potato: Raw potato is an ancient home remedy for backache, characterised by incapacitating pain in the lumbar region, especially in the lower part of the back. Application of raw potato in the form of a poultice has been found very effective in this condition.

Dietary Considerations

The diet of those suffering from backache should consist of a salad of raw vegetables such as tomato, carrot, cabbage, cucumber, radish, lettuce, and, at least, two steamed or lightly-cooked vegetables such as cauliflower, cabbage, carrot, spinach, and plenty of fruits, except bananas. The patient should have four meals daily. Fruit and milk are advised for breakfast, steamed vegetables and wholewheat *chapatis* for lunch; fresh fruit or fruit juice in the evening; and a bowl of raw salad and sprouts during dinner.

The patient should avoid fatty, spicy, and fried foods; curd, sweetmeats and sugar; condiments; and tea and coffee. Foods that have been processed for preservation have few nutrients and should also be eliminated from the diet.

Other Measures

Smoking or taking tobacco in any from should be given up completely. Hot fomentation, alternate sponging, or application of heat to the back will also give immediate relief.

Yogic *asanas* which are beneficial in the treatment of backache are *bhujangasana*, *shalabhasana*, *halasana*, *uttanpadasana* and *shavasana*.

Boils

Local Inflammation of the Skin

Boils are localized, tender, inflamed, pus-filled swellings in the skin surrounded by large red areas. They are infections of the hair follicles of the skin. They are quite painful, particularly in areas where the skin is closely attached to the underlying tissues, such as the nose, ears, or fingers. They usually occur in teenagers and young adults. The common sites for boils are the face, neck, buttocks, and thighs.

Causes and Symptoms

At first, a painful red nodule appears on the skin. This grows bigger and then breaks down in the middle where the pus collects. The patient experiences a great deal of irritation and itching. There may be a single boil, or several boils in the same area or in different areas at or about the same time, or they may come in successive crops. The swelling may not be limited to one hair follicle but may extend to several follicles. When the boils ripen, they give out a discharge. Fever may sometimes accompany the boils.

Boils are caused mainly by *staphylococcus* germs which enter the sweat glands or hair follicles. The essential cause of this disorder is thus bacterial. However, several factors predispose the growth of bacteria in hair follicles. Of these, the chief factor is a toxic condition in the blood stream, which is due to a faulty diet and a frenetic pace of living. Boils generally appear when a person is in a run-down and devitalised condition.

Remedies

Garlic and Onion: Garlic and onions have proved most effective among the several home remedies found beneficial in the treatment of boils. The juice of garlic or onion may be applied externally on boils to help ripen them, break them, and evacuate the pus. An equal quantity of the juices of these two vegetables can also be applied with beneficial results. Eating of two to three pods of garlic during meals will also bring good results.

Bitter Gourd: Bitter gourd is another effective home remedy for blood-filled boils. A cupful of fresh juice of this vegetable, mixed with a teaspoon of lime juice, should be taken, sip by sip, on an empty stomach daily for a few months to treat this condition.

Milk Cream: Milk cream is beneficial in the treatment of boils. One teaspoon of milk cream, mixed with half a teaspoon of vinegar, and a pinch of turmeric powder, makes an excellent poultice. It helps in ripening the blood boils and in their healing without allowing them to become septic.

Betel Leaves: Betel leaves are a valuable remedy for boils. A leaf is gently warmed till it becomes soft. It is then coated with a layer of castor oil. The oiled leaf should be spread over the inflamed part. It should be replaced every few hours. After a few applications, the boil will rupture, draining out all the purulent matter.

Cumin Seeds: Cumin seeds are beneficial in the treatment of boils. The seeds should be ground in water and made into a paste. This paste can be applied to boils with beneficial results.

Margosa Leaves: The use of margosa leaves has proved effective in boils. They can be used as a poultice, decoction, or liniment with beneficial results. To make the decoction, 15 gm of margosa leaves should be boiled in 500 ml of water till it is reduced by one-third.

Parsley: To treat boils, this vegetable should be steeped in boiled water till it is soft and juicy. When comfortably hot, it should be wrapped with clean muslin or linen cloth and applied to the boils as a poultice.

Turmeric: Application of turmeric powder on boils speeds up the healing process. In the case of fresh boils, a few dry roots of turmeric are roasted, the ashes dissolved in a cupful of water, and then applied over the affected portion. This solution enables the boils to ripen and burst.

Dietary Considerations

A thorough cleansing of the system is essential for the treatment of boils. To begin with, the patient may fast on orange juice diluted with water on a 50:50 basis for three to four days, or adopt an exclusive diet of fresh juicy fruits from five to seven days.

After the short juice fast or the all-fruit diet, as the case may be, the patient should adopt a well-balanced diet, with emphasis on wholegrain cereals, raw vegetables, and fresh fruits. Further periods of a juice fast or an all-fruit diet may be necessary, depending on the general health level and bodily condition of the patient.

The patient should avoid tea and coffee, starchy and sugary foods, especially cakes, pastries, sweets, chocolates, white sugar, and white bread. He should also avoid all condiments, pickles, and sauces.

Other Measures

A warm-water enema should be given daily during the initial juice fast or all-fruit diet. This will help to cleanse the bowels. Warm moist compresses should be applied three or four times a day over the tender area. This will help to bring the boil to a head and encourage easy drainage. A hot Epsom salts bath is highly beneficial and should be taken by the patient two or three times in a week until the boils persist and once a week thereafter. Other helpful measures in the treatment of boils are daily dry massage in the morning followed by a cold sponge. Fresh air, breathing exercises, and outdoor exercises are also essential for toning up the system.

In case constipation is habitual, all measures should be taken to overcome it.

Bronchitis

Inflammation of Bronchi

Bronchitis refers to the inflammation of the mucous membrane lining the bronchial tubes within the lungs. Bronchitis may be acute or chronic. In chronic cases, the disease is of long duration and more serious.

Causes and Symptoms

Due to inflammation in the bronchi, large quantities of mucus are secreted and expelled as phlegm. This phlegm is sticky, semi-fluid and may even be purulent. The patient suffers from fever, experiences some difficulty in breathing, and has a cough. Other symptoms are hoarseness, pain in the chest and loss of appetite.

An important cause of bronchitis is smoking. Excessive smoking irritates the bronchial tubes and lowers their resistance, so that they become vulnerable to germs breathed in from the atmosphere. Other causes are living or working in a stuffy atmosphere, use of drugs to suppress earlier diseases, and hereditary factors. Changes in weather and environment hasten the onset of the disease.

Remedies

Turmeric: One of the most effective home remedies for bronchitis is the use of turmeric powder. Half a teaspoon of this powder should be administered with half a glass of milk, two or three times daily. It acts best when taken on an empty stomach.

Ginger: Another effective remedy for bronchitis is a mixture comprising of half a teaspoon each of the powder of ginger, pepper, and cloves, three times a day. It may be licked with honey or taken as an infusion with tea. The mixture of these three ingredients has also antipyretic qualities and is effective in reducing fever accompanying bronchitis. It also tones up the metabolism of the patient.

Onion: Onions have been used as a remedy for bronchitis for centuries. They are said to possess expectorant properties. They liquefy phlegm and prevent its further formation. One teaspoon of raw onion juice, first thing in the morning, is very beneficial in such cases.

Spinach: Fifty grams of fresh leaves of spinach, and 250 ml of water should be mixed with a pinch of ammonium chloride and one teaspoonful of honey. This infusion is an effective expectorant in the treatment of bronchitis.

Sesame Seeds: An infusion of one teaspoon of sesame seeds, mixed with a teaspoon of linseed, a pinch of common salt, and a teaspoon of honey, can be given once at night with beneficial results in bronchitis. Half a teaspoon of dry seeds pounded into powder should be given, mixed with two tablespoons of water, twice daily. Alternately, a decoction of half a teaspoon of the same should be taken twice daily.

Almond: An emulsion of almonds is useful in bronchial diseases, including bronchitis. It is prepared by making a powder of seven kernels of almonds and mixing the powdered kernels in a cup of orange or lemon juice. This emulsion may be taken once daily at night.

Chicory: Chicory or endive is another effective home remedy for bronchitis. The powder of the dry root of this herb should be given in doses of half a teaspoon mixed with one teaspoonful of honey thrice daily. It is a very useful expectorant in chronic bronchitis.

Linseed: A hot poultice of linseed (*alsi*) should be applied over the front and back of the chest. This poultice may be prepared by mixing one cup or sixteen tablespoons of the seeds with a quantity of hot water, sufficient to convert them into a moist mealy mass. This should then be applied carefully. Turpentine may also be rubbed over the chest.

Dietary Considerations

In acute bronchitis, the patient should fast on orange juice and water till the acute symptoms subside. Thereafter, he should adopt an all-fruit diet for two or three days.

In the case of chronic bronchitis, the patient can begin with an all-fruit diet for five to seven days, taking three meals a day of fresh juicy fruits. After the all-fruit diet, he should follow a well-balanced diet with emphasis on seeds, nuts, grains, raw vegetables, and fresh fruits. For drinks, unsweetened lemon water, or cold/hot plain water may be taken.

Other Measures

A hot Epsom salts bath every night or every other night is valuable during the acute stages of the attack. This bath is prepared by dissolving $1\frac{1}{2}$ kg of Epsom salt in 60 litres of water having a temperature of 37.8°C. The patient should remain immersed in the bath for about twenty minutes. In the case of chronic bronchitis, this bath may be taken twice a week.

Hot towels wrung out and applied over the upper chest are helpful in both chronic and acute bronchitis. After applying three hot towels in turn for two or three minutes each, one should always finish off with a cold towel. A cold pack can be applied to the upper chest several times daily in acute conditions. The procedure is to wring out some linen material in cold water, wrap it two or three times round the affected part and cover it with flannel. The pack can remain for about an hour at a time.

Fresh air and outdoor exercise are also essential for the treatment of bronchitis. The patient is advised to take a morning walk every day. He should also perform yogic *kriyas* (cleansing exercises) such as *jalneti* and *vamandhauti*, and yogic *asanas* (body postures) such as *ekpaduttanasana, yogamudra, bhujangasana, shalabhasana, padmasana*, and *shavasana*. Simple *pranayamas* (breath-holding procedures) like *kapalbhati, anuloma-viloma, ujjai*, and *bhramari* will also be beneficial.

Cataract

Opaqueness of the Eye Lens

Cataract is a common eye disease. A cataract refers to an area of the lens of a person's eye that has become whitish and opaque instead of remaining clear. The result is that the person cannot see clearly.

The crystalline lens, through which light travels into the interior of the eye, is situated just behind the iris or coloured portion of the eye. In cataract, this lens becomes opaque, hence, seriously hampering the entrance of light into the eye. Blindness ensues when no light rays can permeate the opacity of the lens.

Causes and Symptoms

The first sign of cataract is blurred vision. The patient finds it difficult to see things in focus. As the disease progresses, the patient may get double vision or spots, or both. At first, vision in twilight may be better than in full daylight since light is admitted round the more widely-dilated pupil in the dark. In the advanced stage, objects and persons may appear as mere blobs of light, and there is a greyish-white discoloration in the pupil.

There are three factors which contribute to the loss of transparency of the lens. These are deterioration in the nutrition of the lens which diminishes the vitality and resistance of the delicate lens fibres; deposits of acids and salts between the lens fibres which have an irritating effect on the lens tissues and exert an increasing pressure on its delicate fibres, gradually destroying them; and disintegration of lens fibres which cloud the entire lens in the absence of appropriate measures.

As in the case of most diseases, poisons in the blood stream due to dietetic errors and a faulty style of living, are the real cause of cataract. The toxic matter in the blood stream spreads throughout the body to find shelter in any available weak spot. It strikes the lens if it has become weak through strain, excessive use of the eyes, and local irritation. The condition becomes worse with the passage of time and then a cataract starts developing. Other causes of cataract are stress and strain; excessive intake of alcoholic drinks, sugar, and salt; smoking; certain physical ailments such as gastro-intestinal or gall-bladder disturbances; diabetes; vitamin deficiencies; fatty acid intolerance; ageing; radiation; side-effects of drugs that have been prescribed for other diseases.

Remedies

Carrot: The use of carrots is considered beneficial in the treatment of cataract. The patient should take plenty of raw carrots daily. As an alternative, he may drink two glasses of fresh carrot juice, one each in the morning and evening.

Garlic: The use of garlic is another effective home remedy for cataract. Two or three cloves should be eaten raw daily. They should be chewed slowly. Garlic helps to clean the crystalline lens of the eye.

Pumpkin: The flowers of pumpkin are valuable in cataract. The juice of these flowers should be extracted and applied externally on the eyelids twice daily. It will stop further clouding of the crystalline lens of the eye.

Aniseed: Aniseed is considered a useful remedy for cataract. An equal quantity of aniseed and coriander powder should be mixed with one teaspoon of brown sugar, and the mixture should be taken in doses of 12 gm in the morning and evening.

Honey: The use of unprocessed pure honey is another effective remedy for cataract. A few drops of this honey should be put in the eyes. This is an ancient Egyptian remedy which has benefitted many patients.

Almonds: Almonds are valuable in cataract. Seven kernels should be ground finely with half a gram of pepper *(kali mirch)* in half a cup of water, and drunk after sweetening the mixture with a teaspoon of sugar candy. It helps the eyes to regain their vigour.

Nutrients: Certain nutrients have also been found useful in cataract. Experiments have shown that animals develop cataract if deprived of pantothenic acid and amino acids, and tryptophane and vitamin B_6 needed for tryptophane assimilation. The diet of the cataract patient should, therefore, be high in vitamins B_2 and B_6, as well as the entire B complex group, pantothenic acid, vitamins C, D, E and other nutrients.

Dietary Considerations

A thorough cleansing of the body is essential. To start with, it will be advisable to undertake a fast of orange juice and water for three days. After this initial fast, a diet of a very restricted nature should be followed for two weeks. Breakfast may consist of seasonal juicy fruits. Raw vegetable salads with olive oil and lemon juice dressing, and soaked raisins, figs, or dates should be taken during lunch. Evening meals should consist of steamed vegetables and a few nuts. Potatoes should be avoided. After two weeks of this diet, the cataract patient may gradually embark upon a well-balanced diet consisting of seeds, nuts, grains, vegetables, and fruits. The emphasis should be on fresh juicy fruits and raw vegetables.

The juice fast followed by the restricted diet should be repeated at an interval of three months. The patient should avoid white bread, sugar, cream, refined cereals, rice, boiled potatoes, puddings and pies, strong tea or coffee, alcoholic beverages, condiments, pickles, and sauces.

Other Measures

A warm-water enema should be given daily during the juice fast. An Epsom salts bath is beneficial and should be taken twice a week. The patient should remain in the bath from twenty-five to thirty-five minutes till he perspires freely. After the bath, he should cool off gradually. Eyes should be closed and bathed externally, at least, twice daily with hot water containing Epsom salts.

Eye exercises aimed at relaxing and strengthening of the eyes are also valuable in cataract The details about these exercises as well as the procedure for palming have been explained in the chapter on Conjunctivitis.

Fresh air and gentle outdoor exercise, such as walking, are other essentials. Exposure to heat and bright light should be avoided.

Chicken Pox

Viral Fever with Rash

Chicken pox is a highly contagious disease, occurring usually in children. It usually affects children of three to four years of age. In most cases, the older the child, the more severe the attack.

Causes and Symptoms

Chicken pox usually begins with a low grade fever, a mild headache and a feeling of weakness. A rash appears on the skin on the first day of the disease. This is in the form of tiny red spots on the skin, mostly on the upper back or chest. In more severe cases, a rash may appear on the face and lower extremities. The papules turn into blisters and finally become pustules and form scabs, which fall off. They come in successive crops, so that while some are drying, others are beginning to form. The skin clears after a few days and the child feels well again. The duration of this disease ranges from ten to twenty-one days but is usually between fourteen and seventeen days.

Chicken pox is caused by a virus. Many researchers believe that the disease is closely related to a much more serious condition known as shingles or herpes zoster that affects adults. The basic cause of the disease, as in most cases of childhood fevers, is however, persistent wrong feeding of children, which results in diminished defence mechanisms of the body.

Remedies

Brown Vinegar: The use of brown vinegar is one of the most important among the several home remedies found beneficial in the treatment of chicken pox. Half a cup of this vinegar should be added to a bath of warm water. This will relieve the irritation of the skin.

Oatmeal: A bath of oatmeal is considered a natural remedy for relieving the itch due to chicken pox. This bath is prepared by cooking two cups of oatmeal in two litres of water for fifteen minutes. This mixture is then put into a cloth bag, preferably cotton, and a string is tied tightly around the top. This bag is allowed to float in a tub of warm water, and swished around until the water becomes turbid. Precaution should be taken to ensure that the bag is not torn. The child with chicken pox can splash and play in the water, making sure that water goes over all the scalds, while the pouch of oatmeal can remain in the tub.

Pea Water: Green pea water is another effective remedy for relieving irritation of the skin. The water in which fresh peas have been cooked can be used for this purpose.

Baking Soda: Baking soda is a popular remedy to control the itching in chicken pox. Some baking soda should be put in a glass of water. The child should be sponged with this water, so that the soda dries on the skin. This will keep the child away from scratching the eruptions.

Vitamin E Oil: The use of vitamin E oil is valuable in chicken pox . This oil should be rubbed on the skin. It will have a healing effect. The marks left by chicken pox will fade away by this application.

Honey: The use of honey as an external application has also proved valuable in chicken pox. The skin should be smeared with honey. It will help in the healing of the disease within three days.

Carrot and Coriander: A soup prepared from carrots and coriander has been found beneficial in the treatment of chicken pox. About 100 gm of carrots and 60 gm of fresh coriander should be cut into small pieces and boiled for a while. The residue should be discarded. This soup should be taken once a day.

Herbal Tea: A mild sedative herbal tea can also prove beneficial in the treatment of chicken pox. This tea can be prepared from any of the herbs like chamomile (*babunah*), basil (*tulsi*), marigold (*zergul*) and lemon balm (*billilotan*). A little cinnamon (*dalchini*), honey, and lemon may be added to this tea. It should be sipped slowly several times a day.

Dietary Considerations

To begin with, the patient should be put on a juice diet for a few days. He should be given plenty of raw fruit and vegetable juices. Lemon juice is considered to be especially beneficial.

As the condition improves, the patient can be placed on an all-fruit diet for the next few days. Thereafter, he may be allowed to gradually adopt a well-balanced diet, with emphasis on fresh fruits and raw vegetables.

Other Measures

A small warm-water enema should be administered daily during the initial juice fast to cleanse the bowels. The patient should be kept in a well-ventilated room. As light has a detrimental effect upon the eyes during an attack of chicken pox because of the weakened condition of the external eye tissues, the patient should shade his eyes from the direct light or the room should have subdued light.

Application of mud packs on the abdomen twice a day, in the morning and evening, and repeated applications of chest packs will be beneficial. Lukewarm water baths can be given every day to relieve itching. For better results, *neem* leaves can be added to this water. The nails of the child should be kept clipped to prevent him from scratching, otherwise, germs on the skin may be scratched into the blisters, causing more severe infection.

Cholera

Watery Motions with Dehydration

Cholera is one of the most severe diseases of the intestines. It is a serious infection involving the lower part of the small bowel. It is a water-borne disease and is common during the monsoon. The mortality rate for this disease has been quite high.

Causes and Symptoms

The first sign of cholera may be mild diarrhoea. This is followed by sudden violent purging. The stools are loose, watery, and greyish-brown in colour. Diarrhoea is usually accompanied by nausea and vomiting. The patient gets severe cramps in the stomach, and feels very thirsty and restless. The temperature rises, but the skin is generally cold and clammy and the pulse is weak. In the next stage, the body becomes colder; the skin dry, wrinkled, and purple; the voice weak and husky; and the urine, scanty and dark. The blood pressure falls, the cramps are agonizing, and signs of collapse appear rapidly.

Cholera is caused by a germ known as *Vibrio cholerae*. This germ produces a powerful poison or endotoxin. The disease is spread by flies and water contaminated by the germs.

Remedies

Lemon: The foremost among the many home remedies for cholera is the use of lemon. The juice of this fruit can kill cholera bacilli within a very short time. It is also a very effective and reliable preventive against cholera during an epidemic. It can be taken in the form of a sweetened or salted beverage for this purpose. Taking of lemon with food as a daily routine can also prevent cholera.

Guava Root Bark: The root bark of guava is rich in tannins and it can be successfully employed as a concentrated decoction in cholera. It arrests vomiting and symptoms of diarrhoea. About thirty grams of the root bark should be used in half a litre of water to make the decoction. The water should be boiled down to reduce it by one-third. This decoction can be taken twice daily.

Onion: Onions are another valuable remedy for cholera. About thirty grams of this vegetable and seven black peppers should be pounded finely in a pestle and given to the patient in two or three doses during the day. Onions allay thirst and restlessness and the patient feels better.

Bitter Gourd: The fresh juice of bitter gourd is an effective medicine in the early stages of cholera. Two teaspoons of this juice, mixed with an equal quantity of white onion juice and a teaspoon of lime juice, should be given twice daily in the treatment of this condition.

Drumstick Leaves: The leaves of the drumstick tree are also useful in this disease. A teaspoon of fresh leaf juice, mixed with one teaspoon of honey and a glass of tender coconut water, can be given two or three times a day as a herbal medicine in the treatment of cholera.

Cucumber: A glass of fresh juice of cucumber leaves with an equal quantity of tender coconut water, given in doses of 30-60 ml, forms a valuable remedy for excessive thirst during cholera. It acts excellently by restoring the acid-base balance in dehydration.

Nutmeg: The herb nutmeg is a valuable remedy for dehydration caused by cholera. An infusion made by steeping half a nutmeg in half a l   of water should be given along with half a litre of tender coconut ater in doses of 15 ml at a time in treating this condition.

Clove: Cloves are useful in cholera. About four grams of this spice should be boiled in three litres of water until half of the water has evaporated. The decoction thus prepared should be given to the patient several times during the day. This will reduce the severe symptoms.

Rough Chaff: The powdered root of rough chaff, botanically known as *Achyranthes aspera*, is also helpful in cholera. About six grams of the powder should be thoroughly mixed with half a cup of water and given to the patient once daily.

Dietary Considerations

The patient should not be given solid food till he has fully recovered from cholera. Liquid bland foods will be easily digested by the patient. Lemon, onions, vinegar, and mint should be included in the daily diet during an epidemic of cholera. All uncooked vegetables should be avoided.

Other Measures

Cholera can be controlled only by rigid purification of water supply and proper disposal of human excreta. In case there is a slightest doubt about contamination of water, it must be boiled before use for drinking and cooking purposes. All foodstuffs must be kept covered, and vegetables and fruits washed with a solution of potassium permanganate before consumption. Those handling food should wash their hands well before starting to cook.

Cirrhosis of the Liver

Cirrhosis of the liver is characterised by a significant loss of cells, so that the liver gradually contracts in size and becomes hard and leathery.

Causes and Symptoms

In the early stages of the disease, there may be nothing more than frequent attacks of indigestion, with occasional nausea and vomiting. There may also be some abdominal pain and loss of weight. In the advanced stage, the patient develops a low grade fever. He has a foul breath, a jaundiced skin and distended veins in the abdomen. Reddish hairlike markings, resembling small spiders, may appear on the face, neck, arms, and trunk. The abdomen becomes bloated and swollen, the mind gets clouded, and there may be considerable bleeding from the stomach.

Excessive use of alcohol over a long period is the most potent cause of cirrhosis of the liver in adults. The disease can progress to the final stage of hepatic failure if the person does not abstain from alcohol. Poor nutrition can be another causative factor in the development of cirrhosis and a chronic alcoholic usually suffers from severe malnutrition. Cirrhosis may also result from a highly toxic condition of the system in general.

Remedies

Papaya Seeds: The black seeds of papaya have been found beneficial in the treatment of cirrhosis of the liver, caused by alcoholism and malnutrition. A tablespoon of juice obtained by grinding the seeds, mixed with ten drops of fresh lime juice, should be given once or twice daily for about a month as a medicine for this disease.

Trailing Eclipta: The herb trailing eclipta, botanically known as *Eclipta alba*, has proved invaluable in cirrhosis of the liver. The juice of all parts of this plant should be taken in doses of one teaspoon, mixed with one teaspoon of honey, three times daily.

Picrorhiza: Picrorhiza, botanically known as *Picrorhiza kurroa*, is a drug of choice in Ayurveda for cirrhosis of the liver among adults. The root of the herb is given in powdered form. A tablespoon

49

of the powder, mixed with an equal quantity of honey, should be administered thrice daily. In case of accompanying constipation, the dose should be increased to double and should be given with a cup of warm water, three to four times a day. It stimulates the liver to produce more bile, the excretion of which relieves congestion of the liver and the tissues.

Vegetable Juices: The juice of carrots, in combination with spinach juice, has been found beneficial in the treatment of cirrhosis of the liver. Spinach juice—200 ml, should be mixed with 300 ml of carrot juice to prepare 500 ml or half a litre of combined juices. Alternatively, 300 ml of carrot juice, combined with 100 ml each of cucumber and beet juices can be used effectively.

Dietary Considerations

The patient must abstain from alcohol in any form. He should undergo an initial liver-cleaning programme by going on a juice fast for seven days. Freshly extracted juices from red beets, lemon, papaya, and grapes may be taken during this period. This may be followed by a fruit and milk diet for two to three weeks. In this regimen, the patient should have three meals a day of fresh juicy fruits such as apples, pears, grapes, grapefruit, oranges, pineapples, and peaches, and a litre of milk divided into three parts, each part to be taken with each fruit meal. The milk should be gradually increased by 250 ml daily and go up to two litres a day. It should be fresh and slightly warmed, if desired. It should be sipped very slowly.

After the fruit and milk diet, the patient should embark upon a well-balanced diet, consisting of seeds, nuts, grains, vegetables, and fruits with emphasis on raw, organically-grown foods. Vegetables such as beets, squashes, bitter gourd, egg-plant, tomatoes, carrots, radishes, and papaya are especially useful in this condition.

All fats and oils should be excluded from the diet for several weeks. The patient should avoid all refined, processed, and canned foods; spices and condiments; strong tea and coffee; fried foods; all preparations cooked in ghee, oil, or butter; all meats; and all chemical additives in food. The use of salt should be restricted.

Other Measures

The patient should be kept in bed. A warm-water enema should be used daily to cleanse the bowels during the juice fast and thereafter, if necessary. Application of hot and cold compresses, for two to three minutes each, on the liver area are beneficial. The morning dry friction, breathing and other exercises should form a regular daily feature of the treatment.

Colitis

Inflammation of the Colon

Colitis refers to inflammation of the colon. The disease results from prolonged irritation and inflammation of the delicate membrane which lines the walls of the colon. Chronic ulcerative colitis is a severe prolonged inflammation of the colon or large bowel, in which ulcers form on the walls of the colon.

Causes and Symptoms

Colitis usually begins in the lower part of the colon and spreads upwards. The first symptom of the trouble is an increased urgency to move the bowel, followed by cramping pains in the abdomen and, sometimes, bloody mucus in the stools. As the disease spreads upward, the stools become watery and more frequent and are characterised by rectal straining. The loss of blood and fluid from the bowels results in weakness, fever, nausea, vomiting, loss of appetite, and anaemia. Other symptoms are a bloated feeling, constipation alternating with diarrhoea or persistent diarrhoea for years together, and insomnia. The patient is usually malnourished and may be severely underweight.

One of the causes of colitis is chronic constipation and the use of purgatives. Constipation causes an accumulation of the hard faecal matter which is never properly evacuated. Purgatives used as a 'cure' only increase irritation. Often colitis results from poorly digested roughage, especially of cereals and carbohydrates, which causes bowel irritation. Other causes of the disease are an allergic sensitivity to certain foods, intake of antibiotics and severe stress.

Remedies

Banana: One or two ripe bananas taken every day are one of the most effective home remedies for ulcerative colitis. Being bland, smooth, easily-digestible and slightly laxative, they relieve the acute symptoms and promote the healing process.

51

Buttermilk: A glass of buttermilk taken daily is another effective remedy for colitis. It is the residual liquid left over after the fat has been removed from curd by churning.

Tender Coconut: Drinking the water of one tender coconut daily has been found valuable in colitis. It is soothing to the soft mucosa of the colon.

Apples: Steamed apples also aid the healing of ulcerative lesions because of their ample concentration of iron and phosphorus.

Drumstick: Drumsticks are also useful in colitis. A teaspoon of fresh leaf juice, mixed with an equal quantity of honey and a glass of tender coconut water, is given two or three times daily as a herbal medicine for the treatment of this disease.

Rice: Rice has a very low fibre content, and is, therefore, extremely soothing in colitis. A thick gruel of rice mixed with a glass of buttermilk and a ripe banana, given twice a day, forms a very nutritious, well-balanced diet in this disease.

Wheat-grass: The juice of wheat-grass (a grass which grows after sowing wheat grains in the earth) used as an enema, helps detoxify the walls of the colon. The general procedure is to first give an enema with lukewarm water. After waiting for twenty minutes, 90–120 ml of wheat-grass juice enema is given. This should be retained for fifteen minutes. This enema is very helpful in disorders associated with colitis. Wheat-grass can be grown at home in earthen pots if it is not available through dealers.

Dietary Considerations

Diet plays an important part in the treatment of colitis. It is advisable to observe a juice fast for five days or so, in most cases of ulcerative colitis. Papaya juice, raw cabbage juice, and carrot juice are especially beneficial. Citrus juices should be avoided.

After the juice fast, the patient should gradually adopt a diet of small, frequent meals of soft cooked or steamed vegetables, rice, porridge, *dalia,* and well-ripened fruits like banana and papaya, yoghurt, and home-made cottage cheese. Sprouted seeds and grains, wholemeal bread, and raw vegetables may be added gradually to this diet after about ten days. All food must be eaten slowly and chewed thoroughly.

Foods which should be excluded from the diet are white sugar, white bread, and white flour products; highly seasoned foods;

highly salted foods; strong tea, coffee, and alcoholic beverages; and foods cooked in aluminium pans.

Other Measures

During the first five days of the juice fast, the bowels should be cleansed daily with a warm-water enema. A buttermilk enema taken twice a week is also soothing and helps in re-installing useful bacterial flora in the colon.

Complete bedrest is very important. The patient should eliminate all causes of tension and face his discomfort with patience.

Common Cold

Viral Throat Infection

A common cold, also known as acute coryza, is an inflammation of the upper respiratory tract caused by infection with common cold viruses. A common cold occurs more often than any other disease — hence, its name. A person may suffer from a common cold several times in a year. A cold usually lasts from three to ten days. The patient feels miserable for the first three days or so.

Causes and Symptoms

The initial signs of a cold are a feeling of soreness of the throat and congestion of the nasal passages. Although the disease normally begins in the nose and throat, it affects all parts of the body. Its usual symptoms are a running nose, sneezing, a rise in temperature, headache, sore throat, chill, aches and pains in the body, and loss of appetite. The skin around the nostrils may become sore.

A common cold results from exposure to the virus. Its intensity, however, depends upon the state of health of the person and environmental factors. Low vitality, exposure to cold, lack of sleep, mental depression, fatigue, and factors such as sudden changes in temperature, dust, and other irritating inhalations are important contributory causes.

Remedies

Lemon: Lemon is the most important among the many home remedies for common cold. It is beneficial in all types of cold with fever. Vitamin C-rich lemon juice increases body resistance, decreases toxicity and reduces the duration of the illness. One lemon should be diluted in a glass of warm water, and a teaspoon of honey should be added to it. This should be taken once or twice daily.

Garlic: Garlic soup is an old remedy to reduce the severity of a cold, and should be taken once daily. The soup can be prepared by boiling three or four cloves of chopped garlic in a cup of water. Garlic contains antiseptic and antispasmodic properties, besides several other medicinal virtues. The oil contained in this vegetable helps to open up the respiratory passages. In soup form, it flushes out all toxins from the system and thus helps bring down fever. Five drops of garlic oil combined with a teaspoon of onion juice, and diluted in a cup of water, should be drunk two to three times a day. This has also been found to be very effective in the treatment of common cold.

Ginger: Ginger is another excellent remedy for colds and coughs. About ten grams of ginger should be cut into small pieces and boiled in a cup of water. It should then be strained and half a teaspoon of sugar added to it. This decoction should be drunk when hot. Ginger tea, prepared by adding a few pieces of ginger into boiled water before adding the tea leaves, is also an effective remedy for colds and for fevers resulting from cold. It may be taken twice daily.

Lady's Fingers: Lady's fingers are highly valuable in treating irritation of the throat and a persistent dry cough. This vegetable is rich in mucilage and acts as a drug to allay irritation, swelling, and pain. About 100 gm of lady's fingers should be cut into pieces, and boiled down in half a litre of water to make a decoction. The steam issuing from this decoction may also be inhaled once or twice a day to relieve throat irritation and a dry cough.

Bitter Gourd Roots: The roots of the bitter gourd plant are used in folk medicine to cure a cold. A teaspoon of the root paste, mixed with an equal quantity of honey or *tulsi* leaf juice, given once every night for a month, acts as an excellent medicine for colds.

Turmeric: Turmeric is an effective remedy for colds and throat irritations. Half a teaspoon of fresh turmeric powder mixed in 30 ml of warm milk, and taken once or twice daily, is a useful prescription for these conditions. Turmeric powder should be put into a hot ladle. Milk should then be poured in it and boiled over a slow fire. This mixture should then be drunk by the patient. In case of a running cold, smoke from the burning turmeric should be inhaled. It will increase the discharge from the nose and provide quick relief.

Tamarind and Pepper: Tamarind-pepper *rasam* is also considered an effective home remedy for a cold in South India. Dilute 50 mg tamarind in 250 ml of water. Boil the diluted tamarind water for a few minutes with a teaspoon of hot ghee and half a teaspoon of black pepper powder. This steaming hot *rasam* has a flushing effect, and should be taken three times a day. As one takes it, the nose and eyes water and the nasal blockage is cleared.

Vitamin C: According to Dr Linus Pauling, a Nobel prize-winning scientist, the regular intake of vitamin C—75 mg for adults and 35 mg for children—will prevent the common cold. If, however, a cold has already appeared, large doses of this vitamin will relieve the symptoms and shorten its duration. He estimates that one to two grams (1000 mg to 2000 mg) per day is approximately the optimum amount of this vitamin for this purpose. His advice is to swallow one or two 500 mg tablets of vitamin C at the appearance of the first sign of the cold and continue the treatment by taking one to two 500 mg tablets daily.

Dietary Considerations

During the acute stage of the cold, when fever is present, the patient should abstain from all solid foods and only drink fruit and vegetable juices, diluted with water. After the acute symptoms are over, the patient can gradually embark upon a well-balanced diet, consisting of seeds, nuts, grains, vegetables, and fruits. It is advisable to avoid meat, fish, eggs, cheese, and starchy foods.

Other Measures

Other useful measures in the treatment of a common cold are a mild sunbath, fresh air and deep breathing, brisk walks, sound sleep, and adjustment of one's clothes and habits to the requirements of the season so as to nullify the effect of weather fluctuations.

Common Fever

Fever refers to a condition of the body in which the temperature goes beyond the normal. It is also characterised by disturbance in the normal functioning of the system. It is a common ailment which occurs both in children and adults.

The average temperature of a healthy body ranges between 36.9^0 C and 37.5^0 C, or 98.4^0 F and 99.5^0 F. It is liable to marginal variations, depending on the intake of food, the amount of exercise, and the temperature surrounding the atmosphere. The lowest temperature of the body occurs between the hours of 1.30 a.m. to 7 a.m. and the highest between 4 p.m. to 9 p.m.

Causes and Symptoms

Fever generally begins with slight shivering, pain in the head and various parts of the body, thirst, and great lassitude. The flow of urine is scanty. As the fever rises, the pulse and respiration become faster. Finally, there is profuse sweating, a copious flow of concentrated urine, and general relief of symptoms.

The term 'fever' has a very wide application. It is the symptom of a body's fight against infection. It is one of the most common features of several diseases. In many cases, it is a secondary symptom of the disordered state of the body with which it is associated. The real cause of all fevers, including common fever, however, is the accumulation of morbid matter in the system due to wrong feeding habits and unhygienic conditions of living. Fever is, thus, a natural attempt on the part of the body to rid itself of toxic matter.

Remedies

Holy Basil: The leaves of holy basil are one of the most effective of several home remedies in the treatment of common fever. A decoction made of about twelve grams of these leaves, boiled in half a litre of water, should be administered twice daily with half a cup of milk, one teaspoon of sugar and a quarter teaspoon of powdered cardamom (*chhoti elaichi*). This will bring down the temperature.

Fenugreek: A tea made from fenugreek seeds is equal in value to quinine in reducing fevers. This tea should be taken twice

56

daily. It is particularly valuable as a cleansing and soothing drink. Fenugreek seeds, when moistened with water, become slightly mucilaginous, and hence, the tea made from them has the power to dissolve a sticky substance like mucus.

Saffron: A tea made from saffron is another effective home remedy for fever. This tea is prepared by putting half a teaspoon of saffron in 30 ml of boiling water. The patient should be given a teaspoon of this tea every hour till the temperature returns to normal.

Raisins: The use of an extract from raisins is beneficial in the treatment of common fever. This extract is prepared by soaking twenty-five raisins in half a cup of water and then crushing them in the same water. They are then strained and the skin is discarded. The raisin water thus prepared becomes a tonic. Half a teaspoon of lime juice added to the extract will enhance its taste and usefulness. It will act as a medicine in fevers, and should be taken twice daily.

Apricot: A cup of fresh juice of apricots mixed with one teaspoon of glucose or honey is a very cooling drink during fevers. It quenches the thirst and eliminates the waste products from the body. It tones up the eyes, stomach, liver, heart, and nerves by supplying vitamins and minerals.

Grapefruit: The juice of grapefruit is a valuable diet in all fevers. It quenches thirst and removes the burning sensation produced by the fever. Half a glass of grapefruit juice should be taken with an equal quantity of water.

Orange: Orange is an excellent food in all types of fever when the digestive power of the body is seriously hampered. The patient suffers from blood poisoning called toxemia, and the lack of saliva results in the coating of his tongue, often destroying his thirst for water as well as his desire for food. The agreeable flavour of orange juice helps greatly in overcoming these drawbacks. Orange juice is the ideal liquid food in fevers. It provides energy, increases urinary output, and promotes body resistance against infections, thereby hastening recovery,

Bloodwort: Bloodwort is one of the best known herbal remedies for fevers. A hot infusion of the herb prepared by steeping 15 gm of the herb in 250 ml of water should be taken twice daily. It will induce perspiration, which will, in turn, cool the fever and expel toxins.

Hog Weed: Another herb found beneficial in the treatment of fever is hog weed. It should be taken twice daily in the form of an infusion prepared by steeping 15 gm of the herb in 250 ml of water. It brings down temperature by inducing copious perspiration.

Dietary Considerations

The patient should be put on a fast of orange juice and water at the beginning of the treatment. The procedure is to drink the juice of an orange in a glass of warm water every two hours from 8 a.m to 8 p.m. After the temperature has come down to normal and the tongue has cleared, the patient may adopt an all-fruit diet for a few more days. In this regimen, he should take three meals a day of fresh juicy fruits. Thereafter, he may gradually embark upon a well-balanced diet according to his age, with emphasis on fresh fruits, and raw or lightly cooked vegetables.

Other Measures

While the patient is on an orange juice fast, a warm-water enema should be given daily to cleanse the bowels. Cold compresses may be applied to the head in case the temperature rises above 39.4^0 C or 103^0 F. If this method does not succeed, a cold pack may be applied to the whole body. The procedure is to wring out a sheet or any other large, square piece of linen material in cold water. It should be wrapped twice right round the body from face downwards. The body should then be covered completely with a thin blanket or similar warm material. This pack should be applied every three hours during the day while the temperature is high, and kept on for an hour or so each time. Hot water bottles may be kept on the feet and against the sides of the body.

Conjunctivitis

Redness of the Eyes

Conjunctivitis refers to an inflammation of the conjunctiva, the thin transparent membrane covering the front of the eye. This is also referred to as having 'sore eyes' and is a very common form of eye trouble. It spreads from person to person through direct contact. Overcrowding, dirty surroundings and unhealthy living conditions can cause epidemics of this ailment.

Causes and Symptoms

The eyeball and underside of the eyelids become inflammed. At first, the eyes are red and itchy. Later, there may be a watery secretion. In more serious cases, there is pus formation, which dries up during sleep, making the lashes stick together.

Conjunctivitis results from bacterial or a virus infection or eye-strain. Prolonged work under artificial light and excessive use of the eyes in one way or the other, no doubt, contribute towards the disease. But its real cause can be traced to a catarrhal condition of the system resulting from general toxaemia due to dietetic errors, and a faulty style of living. The patient generally suffers from colds or other ailments indicative of a general catarrhal condition.

Remedies

A doctor must be consulted before any recommended home remedies are put into the eyes.

Vegetable Juices: Raw juices of certain vegetables, especially carrots and spinach, have been found valuable in conjunctivitis. The combined juices of these two vegetables have proved very effective. In this combination, 200 ml of spinach juice should be mixed with 300 ml of carrot juice. Raw parsley *(prajmoda)* juice—200 ml, mixed with 300 ml of carrot juice has also been found beneficial in the treatment of this disease.

Indian Gooseberry: The juice of the Indian gooseberry, mixed with honey, is useful in conjunctivitis. A cup of this juice should be taken mixed with two teaspoons of honey twice daily in treating this condition.

Vitamins: Vitamins A and B_2 have proved useful in conjunctivitis. The patient should take liberal quantities of natural foods rich in these two vitamins. Foods rich in vitamin A are whole-milk, curds, butter, carrots, pumpkin, green leafy vegetables, tomatoes, mangoes, and papaya. Foods rich in vitamin B_2 are green leafy vegetables, milk, almonds, citrus fruits, bananas, and tomatoes.

Coriander: A decoction prepared with a handful of dried coriander in 60 ml of water is an excellent eye-wash in conjunctivitis. It is said to relieve burning and reduces pain and swelling. This decoction should, however, be sparingly used by persons suffering from bronchial asthma and chronic bronchitis.

Dietary Considerations

The best way to commence treatment for conjunctivitis is to adopt an exclusive fresh fruit diet for a week. In this regimen, the three meals a day should consist of fresh, juicy seasonal fruits. Bananas should, however, not be taken. Those with acute conjunctivitis should undertake a juice fast for three or four days. The short juice fast may be followed by an all-fruit diet for a further seven days. Thereafter, the patient may adopt a restricted diet, consisting of fresh fruits, raw mixed-vegetable salad, wholemeal bread or *chapatis* and steamed vegetables, and nuts.

The patient should avoid an excessive intake of starchy and sugary foods in the form of white bread, refined cereals, potatoes, puddings, sugar, jams, confectionery, meats, fatty foods, strong tea and coffee, too much salt, condiments, and sauces which cause a general catarrhal condition as well as conjunctivitis.

Other Measures

Those taking a juice fast for the first three or four days of the treatment should take a warm-water enema daily during the fast.

A cold water fomentation of the eyes provides almost immediate relief. The procedure is to fold a small hand towel, saturate it with cold water, squeeze out excess water and place the towel gently over both the eyes. It should be covered with a piece of warm cloth to retain the temperature. The process should be repeated as soon as the foment becomes warm. Fomentation should be done for an hour. The eyes should then be covered with a dry towel, and the patient should lie back and relax. The damaged eye tissues will quickly return to normal. This treatment should be repeated every night for a week, even though the problem may clear up with the first treatment itself.

The patient should also adopt various methods of relaxing and strengthening the eyes. These include moving the eyes gently up and down, from side to side and in a circle — clockwise and anticlockwise; rotating the neck in circles and semicircles; and briskly moving the shoulders clockwise and anticlockwise. Palming is highly beneficial in removing strain and relaxing the eyes and its surrounding tissues. The procedure is as follows: sit in a comfortable position and relax with your eyes closed. Cover the eyes with the palms, right palm over the right eye and the left over the left eye. Do not press on the eye balls. Then allow your elbows to drop to your knees, which should be fairly close together.

Constitution

Constipation is a common disturbance of the digestive tract. In this condition, the bowels do not move regularly, or are not completely emptied when they move. This condition is the chief cause of many diseases as it produces toxins which find their way into the bloodstream and are carried to all parts of the body.

Appendicitis, rheumatism, arthritis, high blood pressure, cataract, and cancer are only a few of the diseases in which chronic constipation is an important predisposing factor.

Causes and Symptoms

The most common symptoms of constipation are infrequency, irregularity or difficulty in elimination of the hard faecal matter. The other symptoms include a coated tongue, foul breath, loss of appetite, headache, dizziness, dark circles under the eyes, depression, nausea, pimples on the face, ulcer in the mouth, constant fullness in the abdomen, diarrhoea alternating with constipation, varicose veins, pain in the lumbar region, acidity, heart burn, and insomnia.

The most important causes of chronic constipation are a faulty diet and style of living. Intake of refined and rich foods lacking in vitamins and minerals, insufficient intake of water, consumption of meat in large quantities, excessive use of strong tea and coffee, insufficient chewing, overeating and wrong combination of foods, irregular habits of eating and drinking may all contribute to poor bowel function. Other causes include faulty and irregular habit of defecation, frequent use of purgatives, weakness of abdominal muscles due to sedentary habits, lack of physical activity, and emotional stress and strain.

Remedies

Bael Fruit: Generally all fruits, except banana and jack fruit, are beneficial in the treatment of constipation. Certain fruits are, however, more effective. Bael fruit is regarded as the best of all laxatives. It cleans and tones up the intestines. Its regular use for two or three months throws out even the old accumulated faecal matter. It should be preferably taken in its original form and before dinner. About sixty grams of the fruit are sufficient for an adult.

Pear: Pears are beneficial in the treatment of constipation. Patients suffering from chronic constipation should adopt an exclusive diet of this fruit or its juice for a few days, but in ordinary cases, a medium-sized pear taken after dinner or with breakfast will have the desired effect.

Guava: Guava is another effective remedy for constipation. When eaten with seeds, it provides roughage to the diet and helps in the normal evacuation of the bowels. One or two guavas should be taken everyday.

Grapes: Grapes have proved very beneficial in overcoming constipation. The combination of the properties of the cellulose, sugar, and organic acid in grapes make them a laxative food. Their field of action is not limited to clearing the bowels only. They also tone up the stomach and intestines and relieve the most chronic constipation. One should take at least 350 gm of this fruit daily to achieve the desired results. When fresh grapes are not available, raisins, soaked in water, can be used. Raisins should be soaked for twenty-four to forty-eight hours. This will make them swell to the original size of the grapes. They should be eaten early in the morning, along with the water in which they have been soaked.

Orange: Orange is also beneficial in the treatment of constipation. Taking one or two oranges at bedtime and again on rising in the morning is an excellent way of stimulating the bowels. The general stimulating influence of orange juice excites peristaltic activity and helps prevent the accumulation of food residue in the colon.

Papaya and Figs: Other fruits specific for constipation are papaya and figs. Half a medium-sized papaya should be eaten at breakfast for it to act as a laxative. Both fresh and dry figs have a laxative effect. Four or five dry figs should be soaked overnight in a little water and eaten in the morning.

Spinach: Among the vegetables, spinach has been considered to be the most vital food for the entire digestive tract from time immemorial. Raw spinach contains the finest organic material for the cleansing, reconstruction, and regeneration of the intestinal tract. Raw spinach juice—100 ml, mixed with an equal quantity of water and taken twice daily, will cure the most aggravated cases of constipation within a few days.

Other Remedies: Half a lime, squeezed is a glass of hot water, with half a teaspoon of salt is also an effective remedy for constipation. Drinking water which has been kept overnight in a copper vessel, first thing in the morning, brings good results. Linseed *(alse)* is extremely useful in difficult cases of constipation. A teaspoon of linseed swallowed with water before each meal provides both roughage and lubrication.

Dietary Considerations

The most important factor in curing constipation is a natural and simple diet. This should consist of unrefined foods such as wholegrain cereals, bran, honey, lentils, green and leafy vegetables, fresh and dry fruits, and milk products in the form of butter, ghee, and cream. The diet alone is not enough. Food should be properly chewed. Hurried meals and meals at odd times should be avoided. Sugar and sugary foods should be strictly avoided. Foods which constipate are all products made of white flour, rice, bread, pulses, cakes, pastries, biscuits, cheese, fleshy foods, preserves, white sugar, and hard-boiled eggs.

Other Measures

Toning up the muscles also helps in the treatment of constipation. Fresh air, outdoor games, walking, swimming, and exercise play an important role in strengthening the muscles, and thereby preventing constipation.

Corns

Local Thickening of the Skin

A corn refers to a localized thickening of the skin, especially on the toes, and extending into subcutaneous tissue. A corn is usually small and painful.

Causes and Symptoms

Corns are usually found over the joints of the toes and on the soles of the feet. They are shaped like a pyramid with the apex pointing inwards. They are tender when touched. Sometimes painful and infective warts that occur on the soles of the feet are mistaken for corns.

Corns are usually formed as a result of pressure on the toes and skin surfaces of the feet through incorrect footwear.

Remedies

Liquorice: Liquorice is one of the most valuable remedies for corns that are just appearing. A paste made by grinding three or four liquorice sticks and mixing it with half a teaspoon of sesame oil or mustard oil should be rubbed into the hardened skin at bedtime. The skin gradually softens and the corn decreases in size.

Lemon: Lemon is another valuable remedy for corns. A fresh slice of lemon should be tied over the painful area at night and allowed to remain there the whole night.

Papaya: Raw papaya is beneficial in the treatment of corns. Its juice is an irritant and it is, therefore, a useful application in this condition. Half a teaspoon of raw papaya juice may be applied thrice daily.

Indian Squill: The herb Indian squill, botanically known as *Urginea indica,* is useful in removing corns. A bulb may be roasted and applied over the corn. It should be secured with a bandage. This application may be made at night and removed in the morning.

Green Figs: The milky juice of green figs is valuable for corns of long duration. It helps to soften them. Half a teaspoon of this juice may be extracted from the fruit and applied two or three times daily.

Chalk Powder: Chalk powder has also been found beneficial in the treatment of corns. A small piece of chalk may be ground into a paste with water and applied over the affected area.

Dietary Considerations

A light nutritious diet containing vitamins and minerals in the form of fruits and vegetables is recommended.

Other Measures

For proper treatment of a corn, it is essential to first stop wearing the shoes that caused it. In most cases the corn will disappear when the pressure is removed. Medicinal corn-removing plasters, known as corncaps, are easily available with chemists. They are found to be effective.

For soft corns, which usually occur between the toes, the feet should be washed daily. This should be followed by the application of a mild talcum powder.

Coronary Heart Disease

The term coronary heart disease covers a group of clinical syndromes arising particularly from failure of the coronary arteries to supply sufficient blood to the heart. They include angina pectoris, coronary thrombosis or heart attack, and sudden death without infarction.

Causes and Symptoms

A common symptom of heart disease is shortness of breath, which is caused by the blood being deprived of the proper amount of oxygen. Another common symptom is chest pain or pain down either arm. Other symptoms are palpitations, fainting, emotional instability, cold hands and feet, frequent perspiration, and fatigue.

The basic causes of heart disease are wrong feeding habits, faulty style of living and various stresses. The famous Framingham Heart Study[1] of the National Heart and Lung Institute in Massachusetts, identified seven major risk factors in coronary heart disease. These are: (1) elevated blood levels of cholesterol, triglycerides, and other fatty substances; (2) elevated blood pressure; (3) elevated blood uric acid levels (mainly caused by high protein diet); (4) certain metabolic disorders, notably diabetes; (5) obesity; (6) smoking; and (7) lack of physical exercise. Each or a combination of these risk factors can contribute to heart disease. Most of them are of dietary origin. Constant worry and tension stimulate the adrenal glands to produce more adrenaline and cortisone. This also contributes to constricted arteries, high blood pressure and increased work for the heart.

Remedies

Grapes: Fresh fruits in general are beneficial in the treatment of heart disease. They tone up the heart. Grapes are especially effective in heart pain and palpitation of the heart, and the disease can be rapidly controlled if the patient adopts an exclusive diet of grapes for a few days. Grape juice is particularly valuable when one is actually suffering from a heart attack.

---

1. Linda Clark, *A Handbook of Natural Remedies,* Pocket Books, New York, 1976.

Apple: Apples have heart-stimulating properties. Patients suffering from a weak heart will benefit greatly by making liberal use of this fruit and apple jam.

Indian Gooseberry: Indian gooseberry is considered an effective home remedy for heart disease. It tones up the functions of all the organs of the body, and builds up health by destroying the heterogenous elements and renewing lost energy. When the fruit is in season, one medium-sized Indian gooseberry can be taken with a little salt daily; when not in season, dry pieces can be chewed.

Onion: Onions have been found valuable in heart disease. They are useful in normalising the percentage of blood cholesterol by oxidising excess cholesterol. One teaspoon of raw onion juice first thing in the morning is beneficial in such cases.

Honey: Honey has got marvellous properties to prevent all sorts of heart disease. It tones up the heart and improves the circulation. It is also effective in cardiac pain and palpitation of the heart. One tablespoon daily after food is sufficient to prevent all sorts of heart troubles.

Asparagus: Asparagus is an excellent food for strengthening the heart. A good medicine for a weak or an enlarged heart is prepared by mixing the freshly extracted juice of this vegetable with honey, in the ratio of 2:1. A teaspoon of this medicine should be taken three times daily. Patients with heart disease will also benefit by steam cooking this vegetable.

Alfalfa: The herb alfalfa in the form of juice has been found very helpful in most troubles related to the arteries and heart diseases. Only the leaves of the plant are used for this purpose, when they can be obtained fresh. The juice of fresh alfalfa is, however, too strong and potent to be taken by itself. It is best taken with carrot juice in equal quantities of 125 ml each, twice daily. In this combination, the individual benefits of each juice are intensified.

Safflower: Safflower oil has proved beneficial in lowering blood cholesterol. Hence it can be used liberally with persons suffering from cardiovascular disorders. An emulsion with the trade name Saffloxin-Cipla is used routinely during myocardial infarction, cardiac ischaemia, and hypertension.

Vitamin E: Patients with heart disease should increase their intake of foods rich in vitamin E, as this vitamin is said to promote heart function by improving oxygenation of the cells. It also improves the circulation and muscle strength. Many wholemeal products and green vegetables, particularly outer leaves of cabbage, are good sources of vitamin E.

Vitamin C: Vitamin C is also essential as it protects against spontaneous breaches in capillary walls which can lead to heart attacks. It also guards against high blood cholesterol. The stress of anger, fear, disappointment, and similar emotions can raise blood fat and cholesterol levels immediately but this reaction to stress can do little harm if the diet is adequate in vitamin C and pantothenic acid. One of the richest sources of vitamin C is citrus fruits.

Dietary Considerations

The fundamental conditioning factor in all heart diseases is the diet, which should be lacto-vegetarian, and low on sodium and calories. It should consist of high quality, natural organic foods, with emphasis on wholegrains, seeds, fresh fruits, and vegetables. Foods which should be eliminated from the diet include white flour products, sweets, chocolates, canned foods in syrup, soft drinks, squashes, tea, coffee, alcohol, and tobacco, and all solid fats of animal origin such as butter, cream, and fatty meats. Salt and sugar should be reduced substantially.

Other Measures

The patient should also pay attention to other laws of nature for health building such as taking moderate exercise, getting proper rest and sleep, and adopting a positive mental attitude.

Cough

A Common Symptom of Respiratory Disorders

The air passages of the lungs are lined with cells secreting mucus, which normally traps particles of dust. When the membranes get infected and inflamed, the secretion of mucus increases and the lining of the air passages is irritated. Coughing is the action by which excess mucus is driven out.

Causes and Symptoms

A person who is going to cough first draws a deep breath in. This action causes his glottis to close and his muscles to contract, thus building up pressure in the chest. Then suddenly, the glottis opens, an explosive discharge of air sweeps through the air passages and carries with it the excess secretions or, in some cases, foreign matter, which has irritated the larynx, trachea, or bronchi.

A cough may be caused by inflammation of the larynx or the pharynx. A cough can develop in the chest due to change in weather or seasonal changes. The real cause of this disorder, however, is clogging of the bronchial tubes with waste matter. This is due to wrong feeding habits. The reason for higher incidence of cough during winter than in other seasons is that an average person usually eats more of catarrh-forming foods such as white bread, meat, sugar, porridge, puddings, and pies during the colder months of the year. Being overclothed with heavy undergarments and other garments during this period also prevents proper aeration of the skin.

Remedies

Grapes: Grapes are one of the most effective home remedies for the treatment of a cough. Grapes tone up the lungs and act as an expectorant, relieving a simple cold and cough in a couple of days. A cup of grape juice mixed with a teaspoon of honey is advised for cough relief.

Almonds: Almonds are useful for dry coughs. Seven kernels should be soaked in water overnight and the brown skin removed. They should then be ground well to form a fine paste. A quantity of twenty grams each of butter and sugar should then be added to the paste. This paste should be taken in the morning and evening.

Onion: The use of raw onion is valuable in a cough. This vegetable should be chopped fine and the juice extracted from it. One teaspoon of the juice should then be mixed with one teaspoon of honey and kept for four or five hours—it will make an excellent cough syrup and should be taken twice daily. Onions are also useful in removing phelgm. A medium-sized onion should be crushed, the juice of one lemon added to it, and then one cup of boiling water poured on it. A teaspoon of honey can be added for taste. This remedy should be taken two or three times a day.

Turmeric: The root of the turmeric plant is useful in a dry cough. The root should be roasted and powdered. This powder should be taken in three gram doses twice daily, in the morning and evening.

Belleric Myroblan: The herb belleric myroblan is a household remedy for a cough. A mixture comprising two grams of the pulp of the fruit, 1/4 teaspoon of salt, 1/2 teaspoon of long pepper, and 2 teaspoons of honey should be administered for the treatment of this condition twice daily. The dried fruit covered with wheat flour and roasted, is another popular remedy for cough condition.

Raisins: A sauce prepared from raisins is also useful in a cough. This sauce is prepared by grinding 100 gm of raisins with water. About 100 gm of sugar should be mixed with it and the mixture heated. When the mixture acquires a sauce-like consistency, it should be preserved. Twenty grams should be taken at bedtime daily.

Aniseed: Aniseed is another effective remedy for a hard dry cough with difficult expectoration. It breaks up the mucus. A tea made from this spice should be taken regularly for treating this condition.

Dietary Considerations

In the case of a severe cough, the patient should fast on orange juice and water till the severity is reduced. The procedure is to take the juice of an orange diluted in a cup of warm water, every two hours from 8 a.m. to 8 p.m. After the juice fast, the patient should adopt an all-fruit diet for two or three days. In case of a mild cough, the patient can begin with an all-fruit diet for five to seven days, taking three meals a day of fresh juicy fruits such as apples, pears, grapes, grape-fruit, oranges, pineapples, peaches, and melons. For drinks, unsweetened lemon water, or cold or hot plain water may be given. After the all-fruit diet, the patient should follow a well-balanced diet, with emphasis on wholegrain cereals, raw or lightly cooked vegetables, and fresh fruits.

The patient should avoid meats, sugar, tea, coffee, condiments, pickles, refined and processed foods. He should also avoid soft drinks, candies, ice-cream, and all products made from sugar and white flour.

Other Measures

While the cough is severe, a warm-water enema should be used daily to cleanse the bowels.

Cystitis

Inflammation of the Urinary Bladder

The term 'cystitis' refers to inflammation of the urinary bladder. The recurrence of cystitis may, in some cases, be associated with kidney troubles.

Causes and Symptoms

The patient complains of an almost continual urge to void and a burning sensation on passing urine. There may be a feeling of pain in the pelvis and lower abdomen. The urine may become thick, dark, and stringy. It may have an unpleasant smell and may contain blood or pus. Some pain in the lower back may also be felt in certain cases. In an acute stage, there may be a rise in body temperature. In the chronic form of cystitis, the symptoms are similar but generally less severe and longer lasting, and without a fever.

Cystitis may result from infections in other parts connected with or adjacent to the bladder such as the kidneys, the urethra, the vagina, or the prostate gland. There may be local irritation and inflammation in the bladder if urine is retained there for an unduly long time. Cystitis may also result from severe constipation. Other conditions like an infected kidney, stones in the kidneys or bladder, or an enlarged prostate may also lead to this disorder.

Remedies

Cucumber Juice: Cucumber juice is one of the most useful home remedies in the treatment of cystitis. It is a very effective diuretic. A cup of this juice, mixed with one teaspoon of honey and a tablespoon of fresh lime juice, should be given three times daily.

Drumstick Flowers: Fresh juice of the flowers of drumstick is another effective remedy for cystitis. For better results, a teaspoon of the juice, mixed with half a glass of tender coconut water, should be given twice daily. It acts as a diuretic in the treatment of this disease.

Radish Leaves: The juice of radish leaves is valuable in cystitis. A cup of this juice should be given once daily, in the morning, for a fortnight.

Lady's Fingers: Fresh lady's fingers are useful in cystitis. A decoction made of 100 gm of lady's fingers and 200 ml of water should be taken twice daily in the treatment of this disease.

Spinach: A quantity of 100 ml of fresh spinach juice, taken with an equal quantity of tender coconut water twice a day, is considered beneficial in the treatment of cystitis. It acts as a very effective and safe diuretic due to the combined action of both nitrates and potassium.

Lemon: Lemon has proved valuable in cystitis. A teaspoon of lemon juice should be put in 180 ml of boiling water. It should then be allowed to cool and 60 ml of this water should be taken every two hours from 8 a.m. to 12 noon for the treatment of this condition. This eases the burning sensation and also stops bleeding in cystitis.

Barley: Half a glass each of barley gruel, mixed with buttermilk and the juice of half a lime, is an excellent diuretic. It is beneficial in the treatment of cystitis, and may be taken twice daily.

Sandalwood Oil: The oil of sandalwood is also considered valuable in this disease. This oil should be given in doses of five drops in the beginning and gradually increased to ten to thirty drops. The efficacy of this oil can be increased by the addition of one teaspoon of *ajwain* mixed in a glass of water, or ten grams of ginger mixed in a cup water.

Dietary Considerations

At the onset of acute cystitis, it is essential to withhold all solid foods immediately. If there is fever, the patient should fast on water or tender coconut water for three or four days. If there is no fever, raw vegetable juices, especially carrot juice, should be taken every two or three hours. Half a glass of carrot juice should be mixed with an equal quantity of water and taken at a time. For the next two to three days, only ripe fruits may be taken three or four times daily.

After the all-fruit diet, the patient may gradually embark upon a well-balanced diet, with emphasis on seeds, nuts, grains, vegetables, and fruits. The patient should avoid refined carbohydrates and salt with food and in cooking.

Other Measures

During the first three or four days of acute cystitis, when the patient is on a liquid diet, it is advisable to rest and keep warm. Pain can be relieved by immersing the pelvis in hot water.

Alternatively, heat can be applied to the abdomen, by using a towel wrung out in hot water and covering it with a dry towel to retain warmth. This treatment may be continued for three or four days, by which time the inflammation should have subsided and the temperature returned to normal.

During the next two or three days of an all-fruit diet, cold compresses should be applied to the abdomen. While the hot compresses are intended to relieve pain, the use of cold water compresses is most valuable in relieving pelvic congestion and increasing the activity of the skin. Care should, however, be taken to ensure that compresses do not cause chilling.

Dandruff

Scaliness of the Scalp

The term dandruff generally refers to the condition of the skin wherein shiny, silvery scales separate from the scalp and collect amidst the hair. The condition can become troublesome when the skin gets infected.

Causes and Symptoms

When the hair is combed or brushed, or when the scalp is scratched, the scales from the scalp fall like snowflakes and settle on the eye brows, shoulders, and clothes. These scales sometimes appear as lumps or crusts on the scalp. Often there is itching as well and the scalp may become red from scratching.

The main causes of dandruff are impairment of general health, development of a toxic condition mainly due to taking of wrong foods, constipation, and a low vitality due to infectious diseases. Other factors contributing to this disorder are emotional tension, harsh shampoos, exposure to cold, and general exhaustion.

Remedies

Fenugreek Seeds: The use of fenugreek seeds is one of the most important remedies in the treatment of dandruff. Two tablespoons of these seeds should be soaked overnight in water and ground into a fine paste in the morning. This paste should be applied all over the scalp and left for half an hour. The hair should then be washed thoroughly with soap-nut *(ritha)* solution or *shikakai*.

Lime: The use of a teaspoon of fresh lime juice for the last rinse, while washing the hair, is another useful remedy. This not only leaves the hair glowing but also removes stickiness and prevents dandruff.

Green Gram Powder: A valuable prescription for removal of dandruff is the use of green gram powder. The hair should be washed twice a week with two tablespoons of this powder mixed with half a cup of curd.

Beet: Beets have been found useful in dandruff. Both tops and roots should be boiled in water and this water should be massaged into the scalp with the finger tips every night. White beet is better for this purpose.

Snake Gourd: The juice of snake gourd has been found beneficial in the prevention and treatment of dandruff. The juice should be rubbed over the scalp for this purpose.

Other Remedies: Dandruff can be removed by massaging the hair for half an hour with curd which has been kept in the open for three days, or with a few drops of lime juice mixed with *amla* juice every night, before going to bed. Another measure which helps to counteract dandruff is to dilute cider vinegar with an equal quantity of water and dab this on to the hair with cotton wool in-between shampooing. Cider vinegar added to the final rinsing water after shampooing also helps to disperse dandruff.

Dietary Considerations

Diet plays an important role in the treatment of dandruff. To begin with, the patient should resort to an all-fruit diet for about five days and take three meals a day of juicy fruits. Citrus fruits, bananas, dried, stewed, or tinned fruits should not be taken. After the all-fruit diet, the patient can gradually adopt a well-balanced diet, with emphasis on raw foods, especially fresh fruits and vegetables. Further short periods of an all-fruit diet for three days or so may be necessary at monthly intervals till the skin's condition improves.

Meats, sugar, white flour, strong tea or coffee, condiments, pickles, refined and processed foods should all be avoided.

Other Measures

The foremost consideration in the treatment of this disorder is to keep the hair and scalp clean so as to minimise the accumulation of dead cells. The hair should be brushed daily to improve the circulation and remove any flakiness. The most effective way to brush the hair is to bend forward from the waist with the head down towards the ground, and brush from the nape of the neck towards the top of the head. The scalp should also be thoroughly massaged everyday, using one's finger tips and working systematically over the head. This should be done just before or after brushing the hair. Like brushing, this stimulates the circulation, dislodges dirt and dandruff, and encourages hair growth. Exposure of the head to the rays of the sun is also a useful measure in the treatment of dandruff.

During the first five days of the treatment when the patient takes an all-fruit diet, a warm-water enema should be taken daily to cleanse the bowels. Simultaneously, an attempt should be made to keep the body in good health.

Defective Vision

Myopia, Hypermetropia

Myopia or short-sightedness refers to the inability to see far-off objects clearly. It is a widely prevalent condition.

Causes and Symptoms

Myopia begins with blurred vision, particularly with regard to far-off objects. The blackboard at school, the screen in a cinema hall, or the TV screen may look blurred and the eyes of the sufferer may start watering due to strain. There may be itching and heaviness in the eyes, and the patient may suffer from a mild headache.

The three chief causes of myopia are mental strain, wrong food habits, and improper blood and nerve supply. Mental strain puts a corresponding physical strain on the eyes, and their muscles and nerves. Other causes of this eye disorder are reading in dim light or in too glaring a light; reading in moving trains, buses or cars; watching too much television and films; and excessive reading.

Remedies

Vitamin A: The intake of vitamin A is of utmost importance for improving vision. The best sources of this vitamin are raw spinach, turnip tops, milk cream, cheese, butter, tomatoes, lettuce, carrots, cabbage, soya beans, green peas, fresh milk, oranges, and dates. If taken as a supplement, 25,000 IU of vitamin A are recommended daily.

Triphala: *Triphala*, the famous Ayurvedic preparation, is considered beneficial in the treatment of myopia. This preparation consists of three myrobalans, namely, embelica myrobalan *(amla)*, chebulic myrobalan *(harad)*, and belleric myroblan *(bahera)*. A decoction of this preparation should be made by mixing thirty grams of *Triphala* in half a litre of water and should be taken by mouth and also used for washing the eyes twice a day. This will bring good results if continued for some months.

Liquorice: Another effective remedy for myopia is liquorice. Half a teaspoon of powder of the root, mixed with an equal quantity of honey and half the quantity of ghee, should be given twice daily with a cup of milk on an empty stomach for the treatment of this condition.

Chicory: The herb chicory or endive is extremely valuable in defective vision due to myopia. It contains food elements which are constantly needed by the optic system. It is one of the richest sources of vitamin A which is very useful for the eyes. The addition of juices of carrot, celery, and parsley to chicory juice makes it a highly nourishing food for the optic nerve and the muscular system. It can bring amazing results in correcting eye defects. Half a litre to one litre of this combination, taken daily, has frequently corrected eye troubles in the course of a few months to the extent that normal vision was regained, making the wearing of spectacles unnecessary. The formula proportions considered useful in this combination are 200 ml of carrot juice, 150 ml of celery juice, 75 ml of endive juice and 75 ml of parsley juice to make half a litre of this combination.

Dietary Considerations

Natural, uncooked foods are the best diet for defective vision. These foods include fresh fruits such as oranges, apples, grapes, peaches, plums, cherries; green vegetables like lettuce, cabbage, spinach and turnip tops; root vegetables like potatoes, turnips, carrot, onions, and beetroots; nuts, dried fruits, and dairy products. Cereals are also necessary, but they should only be consumed sparingly. Genuine wholemeal bread is the best and most suitable. Jams, cakes, pastries, white sugar, white bread, confectionery, tea, coffee, meat, fish, and eggs play havoc with the digestion and the body and should therefore be avoided.

Other Measures

A person suffering from defective vision should adopt the various methods of relaxing and strengthening the eyes as outlined in the chapter on Conjunctivitis. Besides these methods, the following measures are also beneficial in the treatment of defective vision:

Sun Gazing: The subject should sit on a bench, facing the rising sun with his eyes closed, and gently sway sideways several times for ten minutes. He should then open his eyes and blink about ten times at the sun and look at some greenery.

Splashing: Plain cold water should be splashed several times over closed eyes. The closed lids should then be rubbed briskly for a minute with a clean towel. This cools the eyes and boosts blood supply.

Swinging: The subject should stand with his feet twelve inches apart, hands held loosely at his sides, his whole body and mind relaxed. He should sway his body from side to side gently, slowly, and steadily, with the heels rising alternately but not the rest of the foot. This movement may be likened to the slow moving of the pendulum of a clock. Swinging should be done in front of a window or a picture, so that the window or picture appears to be moving in the opposite direction of the swing. When facing one end of the window or object, the subject should blink once.

Depression

Feeling Low

Depression is one of the most common emotional disorders. It may be manifested in varying degrees: from feelings of slight sadness to utter misery and dejection. Depression is a very unpleasant malady and is far more difficult to cope with than a physical ailment. The growing complexities of modern life and its resultant crises, as well as the mental stress and strain of day-to-day life, usually leads to this disorder.

Causes and Symptoms

The most striking symptoms of depression are an acute sense of loss, inexplicable sadness, loss of energy, lack of interest in the world around, and fatigue. A disturbed sleep is a frequent occurrence. Other symptoms of depression are loss of appetite, giddiness, itching, nausea, agitation, irritability, impotence or frigidity, constipation, aches and pains all over the body, lack of concentration, and indecisiveness. Cases of severe depression may be characterised by low body temperature, low blood pressure, hot flushes, and shivering.

Prolonged periods of anxiety and tension can cause mental depression. The excessive and indiscriminate use of drugs also leads to faulty assimilation of vitamins and minerals by the body and ultimately causes depression.

Remedies

Apple: Apple is one of the most valuable remedies for mental depression. The various chemical substances present in this fruit such as vitamin B_1, phosphorus, and potassium help the synthesis of glutamic acid, which controls the wear and tear of nerve cells. The fruit should be taken with milk and honey. This remedy will act as a very effective nerve tonic and recharge the nerves with new energy and life.

Cashewnut: The cashewnut is another valuable remedy for general depression and nervous weakness. It is rich in vitamins of the B group, especially thiamine, and is therefore useful in stimulating the appetite and the nervous system. It is also rich in riboflavin which keeps the body active, cheerful, and energetic.

Asparagus: The root of asparagus has been found beneficial in the treatment of depression. It is highly nutritious and is used as a herbal medicine for mental disorders. It is a good tonic for the brain and nerves. One or two grams of the powder of the dry root of the plant can be taken once daily.

Cardamom: The use of cardamom has proved valuable in depression. Powdered seeds should be boiled in water and tea prepared in the usual way. A very pleasing aroma is added to the tea, which can be used as a medicine in the treatment of this condition.

Lemon Balm: The herb lemon balm has been used successfully in the treatment of mental depression. It alleviates brain fatigue, lifts the heart from depression, and raises the spirits.

A cold infusion of the balm taken freely is reputed to be excellent for its calming influence on the nerves. About thirty grams of the herb should be placed in half a litre of cold water and allowed to stand for twelve hours. The infusion should then be strained and taken in small doses throughout the day.

Rose: An infusion of rose petals should be prepared by mixing 15 gm of rose petals in 250 ml of boiling water. If drunk occasionally, instead of the usual tea and coffee, it is beneficial for treating this condition.

Vitamin B: Diet has a profound effect on the mental health of a person. Even a single nutritional deficiency can cause depression in susceptible people. Nutritional therapy builds up brain chemicals, such as serotonin and norepinephrine, that affect the mood and are often lacking in depressed people. Eating foods rich in vitamin B, such as wholegrains, green vegetables, eggs, and fish helps restore vitality and cheer in an individual.

Dietary Considerations

The diet of a person suffering from depression should completely exclude tea, coffee, alcohol, chocolate, colas, all white flour products, sugar, food colourings, chemical additives, white rice, and strong condiments. The diet should be restricted to three meals. Fruits can be taken in the morning for breakfast with milk and a handful of nuts or seeds. Lunch may consist of steamed vegetables, wholewheat *chapatis* and a glass of buttermilk. For dinner, green vegetable salad and all the available sprouts such as alfalfa seeds, moong beans, cottage cheese, or a glass of buttermilk would be ideal.

Other Measures

A person suffering from depression can overcome it by being more active, turning away from himself, and diverting his attention towards other people and things. The pleasure of achieving something overcomes distress or misery. Exercise also plays an important role in the treatment of depression. It not only keeps the body physically and mentally fit, but also provides recreation and mental relaxation. It is nature's best tranquilliser. Exercise also tones up the body, provides a feeling of accomplishment, and reduces the sense of helplessness.

The patient must also learn the art of relaxation and meditation which will go a long way in curing depression. He must gain control over his nervous system and channelise his mental and emotional energies into restful activities. This can be achieved by ensuring sufficient rest and sleep under quiet conditions. Meditation will help create a balance in the nervous system. This will enable the hormonal glands to return to a correct state of hormonal balance and thereby overcome the feeling of depression.

Diabetes Mellitus

Diabetes mellitus is characterised by an abnormally high level of blood glucose and by the excretion of the excess glucose in the urine. It results from an absolute or relative lack of insulin which leads to abnormalities in carbohydrate metabolism as well as in the metabolism of protein and fat.

The most commonly-used screening tests are the determination of the fasting blood glucose level and the blood glucose level tested two hours after a meal. The normal fasting blood sugar content is 80—120 mg per 100 ml of blood; this can go up to a level of 160 mg per 100 ml of blood two hours after meals. Anything above these levels can be termed as diabetic levels. Diabetes is common among older, obese people.

Causes and Symptoms

A diabetic feels hungry and thirsty most of the time, does not put on weight, and gets tired easily, both physically and mentally. He looks pale, and may suffer from anaemia, constipation, intense itching around the genital organs, palpitations, and general weakness. He feels drowsy and has a lower sex urge than a normal person.

Diabetes has been described as a prosperity disease, primarily caused by overeating and consequent obesity. Not only is the overeating of sugar and refined carbohydrates harmful, but an excessive intake of proteins and fats, which are transformed into sugar if taken in excess, may also result in diabetes. Grief, worry, and anxiety also have a deep influence on the metabolism and may cause sugar to appear in the urine.

Remedies

Bitter Gourd: Among the several home remedies that have proved beneficial in controlling diabetes, perhaps the most important is the use of bitter gourd. It has lately been established that bitter gourd contains a hypoglycaemic or insulin-like principle, designated as 'plantinsulin', which has been found valuable in lowering the blood and urine sugar levels. It should, therefore, be included liberally in the diet of the diabetic. For better results, the diabetic should take the juice of about four or five *karelas* every morning on an empty stomach. The seeds can be added to food in a powdered form. Diabetics can also use bitter gourd in the form of a decoction by boiling the pieces in water or in the form of dry powder.

Indian Gooseberry: Indian gooseberry, with its high vitamin C content, is considered valuable in diabetes. A tablespoon of its juice, mixed with a cup of bitter gourd juice, taken daily for two months, will stimulate the islets of Langerhans, that is, the isolated group of cells that secrete the hormone insulin in the pancreas. This mixture reduces the blood sugar in diabetes.

Jambul Fruit: Jambul fruit is another effective home remedy. It is regarded in traditional medicine as a specific against diabetes because of its effect on the pancreas. The fruit as such, the seeds, and fruit juice are all useful in the treatment of this disease. The seeds contain a glucoside 'jamboline' which is believed to have the power to check the pathological conversion of starch into sugar in cases of increased production of glucose. The seeds should be dried and powdered. One teaspoon of this powder should be mixed in one cup of milk or water or half a cup of curd, and taken twice daily.

The inner bark of the jambul tree is also used in the treatment of diabetes. The bark is dried and burnt. It will produce an ash of white colour. This ash should be pestled in mortar, strained and bottled. The diabetic patient should be given ten grams of this ash on an empty stomach with water in the morning, and twenty grams in the afternoon, and in the evening an hour after taking meals.

An equal quantity of *amla* powder, *jamun* powder, and bitter gourd powder also makes a very useful remedy for diabetes. A teaspoon of this mixture once or twice a day would be effective in checking the progress of the disease.

Grapefruit: According to Dr Joe Shelby Riley, a well-known expert in nutrition, 'Grapefruit is a splendid food in the diet of a diabetic patient. If grapefruits were eaten more liberally, there would be much less diabetes. If you have sugar, use three grapefruits three times a day. If you do not have sugar, but a tendency towards it and want to prevent it, use three a day."[1]

Fenugreek: The seeds of fenugreek have been found effective in the treatment of diabetes. Fenugreek seeds, when given in varying doses of 25 gm to 100 gm daily, diminish reactive hyperglycaemia in diabetic patients. Levels of glucose, serum cholesterol, and triglycerides were also significantly reduced in the diabetes patients when the seeds were consumed.

Bengal Gram: Experiments have shown that the intake of water extract of Bengal gram enhances the utilization of glucose in both diabetic and normal persons. Tests were conducted at the Central Food Technological Research Institute in Mysore on a chronic diabetes patient whose insulin requirement was of the order of forty units a day. When kept on a diet which included liberal supplements of Bengal gram extract, the condition of the patient improved considerably and his insulin requirement was reduced to about twenty units per day. Diabetes patients who are on a prescribed diet which does not severely restrict the intake of carbohydrates, but includes liberal amounts of Bengal gram extract, have shown considerable improvement in their fasting blood sugar levels, glucose tolerance, urinary excretion of sugar, and general condition.

Black Gram: For a milder type of diabetes, two tablespoons of germinated black gram, taken with half a cup of fresh bitter gourd juice and a teaspoon of honey, is said to be useful. It should be taken once daily for three to four months. A restriction should be placed on the intake of carbohydrates. Even in severe cases, regular use of this combination, with other precautions, is useful as a health-giving food for the prevention of various complications that may arise due to malnutrition in diabetics.

Mango Leaves: The tender leaves of the mango tree are considered useful in diabetes. An infusion is prepared by soaking 15 gm of fresh leaves in 250 ml of water overnight, and squeezing them well in the water in the morning. This filtrate should be taken every morning to control early diabetes. As an alternative, the leaves should be dried in the shade, powdered and preserved for

---

1. Dr S.J. Singh, *Food Remedies*, 4th edition, Nature Cure Council of Medical Research, Lucknow, 1982.

use when necessary. Half a teaspoon of this powder should be taken twice a day. If you do not have sugar, but...

Parslane: The seeds of parslane are useful in diabetes. A teaspoon of the seeds should be taken every day with half a cup of water for three to four months. It will increase the body's own insulin and help in curing diabetes.

Other Foods: Besides bitter gourd, certain other vegetables have been found useful in diabetes. These include string beans, cucumber, onion, and garlic. Tea made of the pods of string beans is valuable in diabetes.

Dietary Considerations

The primary dietary consideration for a diabetic is that he should be a strict lacto-vegetarian and take a low-calorie, low-fat, alkaline diet of high-quality natural foods. Wholegrains, fruits, nuts, vegetables, and dairy products form a good diet for the diabetic. Emphasis should be on raw foods as they stimulate the pancreas and increase insulin production. Home-made cottage cheese and various forms of soured milk such as curd and buttermilk are the best sources of proteins.

Other Measures

Exercise is also an important factor in the treatment of diabetes. Light games, jogging, and swimming are recommended. Yogic *asanas* such as *bhujangasana, shalabhasana, dhanurasana, paschimottanasana, sarvangasana, halasana,* and *shavasana* will be beneficial.

Diarrhoea

Diarrhoea refers to the frequent passage of loose or watery unformed stools.

Causes and Symptoms

Diarrhoea may be acute or chronic. Commonly known as 'loose motions', it is one of the commonest diseases, particularly in India, in children.

The small intestine normally gets more than ten litres of liquid per day which comes from the diet and from secretions of the stomach, liver, pancreas, and intestines. In the case of diarrhoea, water is either not absorbed or is excreted in excess. It is then sent to the colon whose water-holding capacity is limited. Thus the urge to defecate comes quite often.

The main causes of diarrhoea are overeating or eating of wrong foods, putrefaction of food in the intestinal tract, fermentation caused by incomplete carbohydrate digestion, nervous irritability, use of antibiotic drugs, and excessive intake of laxatives. Other causes include parasites, germs, virus, bacteria, or a poison which has entered into the body through food, water, or air; allergies to certain substances or even common foods such as milk, wheat, eggs, and sea foods; emotional strain or stress in adults and fright in children. Certain organic diseases affecting the intestines may also lead to diarrhoea.

Remedies

Buttermilk: Buttermilk is one of the most effective home remedies in the treatment of diarrhoea. Buttermilk is the residual milk left after the fat has been removed from curd by churning. It helps overcome harmful intestinal flora. The acid in the buttermilk also fights germs and bacteria. Buttermilk may be taken with a pinch of salt three or four times a day for controlling this disease.

Carrot Soup: Carrot soup is another effective home remedy for diarrhoea. It supplies water to combat dehydration; replenishes sodium, potassium, phosphorus, calcium, sulphur, and magnesium; supplies pectin; and coats the intestine to allay inflammation. It also checks the growth of harmful intestinal bacteria and prevents vomiting. Half a kilogram of carrots may be cooked in 150 ml of water until they become soft. The pulp should be strained and enough boiled water added to it to make a litre. Three-quarters of a tablespoon of salt may be added. This soup should be given in small amounts to the patient every half an hour.

Fenugreek: Fenugreek leaves are useful in diarrhoea. One teaspoon of seeds which have been boiled and fried in butter should be taken with a cup of buttermilk twice daily. They are valuable in allaying biliousness. The seeds are also beneficial in the treatment of this disease.

Ginger: In case of diarrhoea caused by indigestion, dry or fresh ginger is very useful. A piece of dry ginger should be powdered along with a crystal of rock salt, and quarter of a teaspoon of this powder should be taken with a small piece of jaggery. It will bring quick relief as ginger, being carminative, aids digestion by stimulating the gastrointestinal tract.

Mint: Mint juice is also beneficial in the treatment of diarrhoea. One teaspoon of fresh mint juice, mixed with a teaspoon each of lime juice and honey, can be given thrice daily with excellent results in the treatment of this disease.

Bottle Gourd: The juice of bottle gourd is a valuable medicine for excessive thirst due to severe diarrhoea. A glass of plain juice with a pinch of salt should be taken every day in treating this condition.

Drumstick Leaves: The juice of fresh leaves of drumstick is also valuable in diarrhoea. A teaspoon of this juice, mixed with a teaspoon of honey and a glass of tender coconut water, can be given two to three times as a herbal medicine in the treatment of diarrhoea.

Pomegranate: The pomegranate has proved beneficial in the treatment of diarrhoea on account of its astringent properties. If the patient develops weakness due to profuse and continuous purging, he should repeatedly be given about 50 ml of pomegranate juice to drink. This will control the diarrhoea.

Mango Seeds: Mango seeds are valuable in diarrhoea. The seeds should be collected during the mango season, dried in the shade and powdered, and kept stored for use as a medicine when required. A dose of about one and a half to two grams with or without honey, should be administered twice daily.

Sesame Seeds: Sesame seeds are helpful in the treatment of this condition. Two tablespoons of the seeds should be lightly roasted in a frying pan. They should then be ground into a fine powder and mixed with one tablespoon of cow's ghee. The mass should be divided into three parts and each part should be taken with half a cup of boiled goat's milk thrice daily for six days by the patients. It acts as an excellent medicine in this condition.

Turmeric: Turmeric has proved to be another valuable home remedy for diarrhoea. It is a very useful intestinal antiseptic. It is also a gastric stimulant and tonic. One teaspoon of fresh turmeric rhizome juice or one teaspoon of dry rhizome powder may be taken in one cup of buttermilk or plain water.

Rice: Rice is useful in treating diarrhoea in children. A teaspoon of powder of charred parboiled rice, mixed with a glass of buttermilk, should be given in doses of thirty grams every half an hour. This will bring excellent results.

Other Remedies: Cooked or baked apples are good for diarrhoea. The cooking process softens the cellulose. Much of its value as a regulating material is thus lost and it is effective in looseness of the bowels.

A glass of fresh tomato juice, mixed with a pinch of salt and pepper, taken in the morning, also proves beneficial.

Other starchy liquids such as arrowroot water, barley water, and coconut water are also useful in the treatment of diarrhoea. They not only replace the fluid lost but also bind the stools. Other home remedies include bananas and garlic. Bananas contain pectin and encourage the growth of beneficial bacteria. Garlic is a powerful, effective, and harmless germ killer. It aids digestion and removes intestinal worms.

Dietary Considerations

In severe cases of diarrhoea, it is advisable to observe a complete fast for two days to provide rest to the gastrointestinal tract. Only hot water may be taken during this period to compensate for the loss of fluids. Juices of fruits may be taken after the acute symptoms are over. After the condition improves, meals can be enlarged gradually to include cooked vegetables, whole rice, soured milk. Raw foods should be taken only after the patient completely recovers.

Other Measures

Other useful methods for the treatment of diarrhoea are the application of cold compress at 15.6^0C on the abdomen and a cold hip bath at 4.5^0C–10^0C. The procedure for cold compress is to wring a folded cloth from cold water and apply it on the abdomen. The wringing should be just sufficient to prevent dripping. The compress should be renewed every fifteen to twenty minutes. For a cold hip bath, a special type of bath tub is used. It is filled with cold water so that it covers the hip and reaches up to the level where the patient's navel is covered in a sitting position. The duration of the bath is usually ten to fifteen minutes. The patient should rub the abdomen from the naval downwards in brisk anticlockwise movements across the body with a moderately coarse, wet cloth. The legs, feet, and upper part of the body should remain completely dry during and after the bath.

Dropsy

Dropsy, technically known as oedema, refers to the abnormal accumulation of fluid in the body. It may be general or localized.

Causes and Symptoms

In the case of kidney disease, dropsy is first noticed beneath the eyes and face, and is worse in the mornings. In the case of heart disease, the swelling tends to be worse in the evenings and begins in the lower parts of the body such as the ankles. In liver disease, which is often the result of chronic alcoholism, the swelling is in the legs and abdomen. Oedema occurs in many diseases, especially those relating to the heart, kidney, and liver.

Remedies

Pineapple: Pineapple is one of the many home remedies found beneficial in the treatment of dropsy. It contains sufficient chlorine which stimulates the activity of the kidneys and helps remove much of the waste products from the body. It also relieves the body of a waterlogged condition.

Arjuna: Another effective remedy for dropsy is the use of the herb *arjuna*. This herb has been employed successfully by practitioners of the indigenous system of medicine in the treatment of this condition. Thirty grams of the thick bark can be mixed with 250 ml of milk to make a decoction, and taken every morning on an empty stomach.

Alternately, one or two grams of the powder of the bark can be added to a cup of milk with sufficient jaggery to sweeten it, and taken every morning on an empty stomach.

Indian Squill: Another remedy found valuable in dropsy is the herb Indian squill. It has diuretic properties and increases the secretion and discharge of urine. The bulb of the herb should be sliced and used in a small quantity of twenty to thirty grams.

Black Nightshade: Black nightshade has proved beneficial in the treatment of dropsy. It can be taken both in the form of a decoction or as a vegetable. The decoction can be made by boiling thirty grams of black nightshade in half a litre of water, till it is reduced by one-third. This can be taken twice daily. An extract of the leaves and stem, in doses of 6 - 8 ml can also be taken twice daily.

Lime Water: Lime water has also proved effective in the treatment of this condition. The whole belly should be covered with a large, absorbant towel, which has been dipped in strong lime water and then squeezed out.

Dietary Considerations

To begin with, the patient should fast on fruit and vegetable juices for about five days. He should take a glass of juice diluted with water on a 50:50 ratio during this period. After the juice fast, he may spend another three or four days on an exclusive fruit diet, taking three meals a day of juicy fruits such as apples, grapes, pineapple, and papaya at five-hourly intervals. Thereafter he may gradually embark upon a well-balanced diet, with emphasis on fresh fruits and raw vegetables.

Other Measures

The patient is advised to take a warm-water enema daily during the juice fast and the all-fruit diet. This will help immensely in cleansing the bowels. A hot water bath taken daily will also be beneficial in the treatment of dropsy.

Dysentery

Bloody Loose Motions

Dysentery is a serious condition affecting the large intestine. The pathological condition of this disease is caused by two organisms, protozoa and bacilli. When caused by the former, the condition is generally known as amoebic dysentery, and when caused by the latter, it is known as bacillary dysentery.

Causes and Symptoms

Dysentery may be acute or chronic. The acute form is characterised by pain in the abdomen and diarrhoea. Yellowish-white mucus and, sometimes, only blood from the intestinal ulcers is passed with the stools. The evacuations are preceded by pain and tenesmus. The patient feels a constant desire to evacuate, although there may be nothing to throw off except a little mucus and blood. Chronic cases are after-effects of acute attacks. In severe cases, the temperature may rise to 40^0C — 40.6^0C. It may occasionally become subnormal also.

The cause of dysentery, according to the modern medical system, is germ infection. The germs, which are supposed to cause dysentery, only develop in the colon as a result of putrefaction of excessive quantities of animal protein food, fried substances, spicy foods, and hard-to-digest fatty substances. The real cause of dysentery is, thus, dietary indiscretion and eating of excessive amounts of flesh foods in hot weather or tropical climate unsuited to the digestion of such foods. Other causes include debility, fatigue, chill, lowered vitality, intestinal disorders, and overcrowding under insanitary conditions.

Remedies

Bael Fruit: Among specific home remedies, bael fruit is perhaps the most efficacious in the treatment of dysentery of both varieties. One tablespoon of the pulp of the fruit, mixed with a sufficient quantity of jaggery to sweeten it, should be given thrice daily. To deal with a chronic case of dysentery, 15 gm of the unripe fruit pulp should be roasted over the fire and the pulp mixed with 250 ml of water or buttermilk. Just enough jaggery to sweeten the infusion should be added, and the infusion should be taken thrice daily. Fifteen grams of the pulp of the unripe fruit mixed with an equal quantity of dried ginger, can also be given with 250 ml of buttermilk, thrice daily.

Pomegranate Rind: The use of pomegranate rind is another effective remedy for dysentery. About 60 gm of the rind should be boiled in 250 ml of milk. It should be removed from the fire when one-third of the milk has evaporated, and then be administered to the patient in three equal doses at suitable intervals. This will relieve the disease very soon.

Lemon: Lemon juice is very effective in dealing with ordinary cases of dysentery. Three lemons, peeled and sliced, should be added to 250 ml of water and boiled for a few minutes. The strained infusion should be administered thrice daily.

Musk Melon: Musk melon is useful in dysentery which is often accompanied by a soft and mucilaginous secretion in the intestines, leaving some of its portion stuck up within. If this condition persists for a long time, it forces the intestines to contract.

This fruit is endowed with remarkable qualities to expel this nasty matter with faeces.

Ribbed Gourd Seeds: The seeds of ribbed gourd contain a chemical similar to emetine and, hence, they can be effectively used in acute and chronic amoebic dysentery. About five to ten grams of the seeds can be given with one cup of buttermilk twice daily with beneficial results in amoebic dysentery.

Ishabgul: The seeds of this herb are very useful in several kinds of chronic dysentery. In case of heaviness in the stomach and the intestines in dysentery, about 50 ml of castor oil should be administered with one cup of milk thrice daily, to eject hard lumps of stools. After a few motions have cleared the intestine, 10 gm of ishabgul seeds, mixed with about 100 gm of curd, should be taken three to four times a day.

Other Remedies: Other remedies considered useful in the treatment of dysentery are small pieces of onion mixed with curd and equal parts of the tender leaves of the peepal tree, coriander leaves, and sugar, chewed slowly.

Dietary Considerations

To begin with, the patient should fast as long as acute symptoms are present. Only orange juice and water should be taken during this period. As an alternative, the patient should subsist on buttermilk till the acute symptoms are over. Buttermilk combats offending bacteria and helps establishment of benign micro-organisms in the intestines.

After the acute symptoms are over, the patient may be allowed rice, curd, fresh ripe fruits, and skimmed milk. Solid foods should be introduced very carefully and gradually according to the pace of recovery. Flesh foods of all kinds should be avoided. Other foods which should be avoided are tea, coffee, white sugar and white flour, and alcohol in all forms.

Other Measures

The patient may be given small doses of castor oil in the form of an emulsion. This acts as a mild laxative and facilitates quick removal of offensive matter, minimises the strain during defecation, and also acts as a lubricant on the ulcerated surfaces. The mechanical removal of accumulated poisonous matter should also be attempted by giving very low pressure enema, twice or thrice daily, admitting as much water as the patient can tolerate. A hot water bag may be applied over the abdomen.

Dyspepsia

Dyspepsia is a word of Greek origin meaning indigestion or difficulty in digestion. It is a common ailment and results from dietetic errors.

Causes and Symptoms

Abdominal pain, a feeling of undue fullness after eating, heartburn, loss of appetite, nausea or vomiting, and flatulence or gas are the usual symptoms of dyspepsia. Vomiting usually provides relief. What is vomited is intensely sour to the taste. Other symptoms are a foul taste in the mouth, coated tongue, and foul breath. At times a sensation of strangling in the throat is experienced. In most cases of indigestion, the patient suffers from constipation.

The main causes of dyspepsia are overeating, eating wrong food combinations, eating too rapidly, and neglecting proper mastication and salivation of food. Overeating makes the work of the stomach, liver, kidneys, and bowels harder. When the food putrefies, its poisons are absorbed into the blood and, consequently, the whole system is poisoned. Certain foods, especially if they are not properly cooked, cause dyspepsia. Other causes are intake of fried food, rich and spicy foods; excessive smoking; intake of alcohol; constipation; habit of eating and drinking together; insomnia; emotions such as jealousy, fear, and anger; and lack of exercise.

Remedies

Lemon: The use of fruits in general is beneficial in the treatment of dyspepsia. They flush out the undigested food residue and accumulated faeces, and re-establish health to perfect order. The best fruit for the treatment of dyspepsia is lemon. Its juice reaches the stomach and attacks the bacteria, inhibiting the formation of acids. Lemon juice removes indigestion by dislodging this acid and other harmful substances from the stomach, thereby strengthening and promoting a healthy appetite. The juice of one lemon, diluted with water, can be taken twice daily before each principal meal.

Grapes: The use of grapes is another effective remedy for dyspepsia. This fruit is a light food and removes indigestion and irritation of the stomach in a short time. About 250 gm can be taken daily.

Pineapple: Another fruit useful in dyspepsia is pineapple. It acts as a tonic and relieves much of the digestive disorders of the dyspeptics. Half a glass of pineapple juice should be taken after one meal in treating this condition.

Pomegranate: One tablespoon of pomegranate juice, mixed with a tablespoon of honey, is valuable in indigestion accompanied by giddiness. This dose may be taken twice daily. The seeds of this fruit act as a stomach tonic when mixed with a little rock salt and black pepper powder.

Carrot: Carrots are valuable in dyspepsia. Chewing of this vegetable increases saliva and quickens digestion by supplying the necessary enzymes, minerals, and vitamins. Half a glass of carrot juice, diluted with an equal quantity of water, can be taken once daily to treat this disorder.

Fenugreek: Fenugreek leaves are beneficial in dyspepsia. About fifty grams of leaves, boiled and fried in butter, are valuable in allaying biliousness. The seeds can also be used beneficially in the treatment of dyspepsia.

Mint: Mint is also very useful in correcting dyspepsia because of its digestive properties. Mint juice is a good appetiser. One teaspoon of mint juice, mixed with an equal amount of honey and lemon juice, forms a very effective remedy for indigestion and gaseous distension of the stomach.

Buttermilk: A very simple remedy for indigestion is a glass of thin buttermilk mixed with a quarter teaspoon of pepper powder. For better results an equal quantity of cumin powder may be added to the buttermilk.

Aniseed: The use of aniseed is also beneficial in the treatment of indigestion. An infusion can be prepared by mixing a teaspoon of aniseed in a cup of boiling water and leaving it covered overnight. The clear fluid can then be decanted and taken with honey.

Dietary Considerations

The best way to commence treatment is to adopt an all-fruit diet for five days. The patient may, thereafter, gradually embark upon a well-balanced diet, consisting of fresh fruits, raw and steamed vegetables, seeds, nuts, and whole grains.

Other Measures

The patients suffering from indigestion must always follow

91

certain rules regarding eating. These include not eating and drinking together; never to hurry through a meal; never to eat on a full stomach; never to sit down to a meal when worried, tired, excited, or in a bad temper; and not to eat if an appetite is lacking.

Earache

Pain in the Ear

Earache is a common disorder, resulting either from infection in the outer ear canal or the middle ear.

Causes and Symptoms

Outer ear canal infection is common in summer during the swimming season, and can be localised as an itchy, foul-smelling, painful boil or furuncle. Middle ear infection is more common in very young children, and may be accompanied by high fever, nausea, vomiting, and diarrhoea.

Remedies

Garlic: The use of garlic has been found beneficial in the treatment of earache. Three cloves should be warmed and mashed with a pinch of salt. This mixture should be wrapped in a piece of woollen cloth and placed on the painful ear. Simultaneously, two or three cloves of garlic should be chewed daily for a few days. This will give relief.

Garlic oil is also a popular remedy for earache. If garlic oil is not available, a few peeled cloves of garlic can be put in a tablespoon of any sweet oil, except groundnut oil. This oil should be heated, till the oil becomes brown and the garlic pieces charred. The oil should then be filtered and cooled, and a few drops should be put into the affected ear. This will give immediate relief.

Marigold: The leaves of this flower are another effective home remedy for earache. These leaves should be warmed and the lukewarm juice of these leaves should be extracted. Two or three drops of this juice can be put in the affected ear with gratifying results.

Holy Basil: The leaves of holy basil are considered beneficial in the treatment of earache. The juice of these leaves should be extracted and two or three drops put in the ear for relieving the pain.

Alkanet Root: The herb alkanet root is commonly available in a grocer's shop. Boiled in mustard oil, it makes an effective medicine for earache. About 125 gm of black mustard oil should be boiled in a tin basin on a gentle fire. Then twelve grams of alkanet root should be put in this oil and allowed to burn in it. The oil should be filtered when cooled and filled in a bottle. Two or three drops of this oil should be put in the ear in case of emergency. This will give great relief.

Dhatura Leaves: The juice of the leaves of the dhatura plant boiled in sesame (*til*) oil can also be used beneficially as a medicine for earache. About 25 ml each of the juice of dhatura leaves and sesame oil should be boiled in a tin basin on a gentle fire. When half the juice remains, about seven leaves of gigantic swallow wart *(AK)*, smeared with sesame oil and sprinkled with powdered salt, should also be put in this oil. It should be boiled till the leaves are burnt. The oil should, thereafter, be filtered through a coarse cloth and preserved safely in a bottle. A few drops of this oil dropped in the ear will cure the earache.

Bishop's Weed: This herb is beneficial for an earache. About half a teaspoon of the seeds is heated in 30 ml of milk, till the essence of the seeds permeates the milk. The milk is then filtered and used as ear-drops. Two or three drops put twice daily will decrease congestion and relieve pain.

Cloves: A clove should be sauted in a teaspoon of sesame (*til*) oil, and three to five drops of this warm oil should be put into the affected ear two or three times daily. This will provide relief.

Dietary Considerations

The person suffering from earache should take an all-fruit diet for three to five days. After that, a well-balanced diet comprising wholegrain cereals, raw or highly-cooked vegetables, and fresh fruits may be taken. White flour and sugar and their products, pickles, condiments, and flesh foods should be avoided, along with food which raise the amount of phlegm, such as milled rice, sugar, and lentils.

Other Measures

During the all-fruit diet, a warm-water enema should be used daily to cleanse the system. Regular exercises, outdoor games, and fresh air are important. The patient should sit in the sun and allow the sunlight to penetrate the inner part of his ear for fifteen minutes. This will stop the discharge of pus from the ear.

Ear Discharge

Pus from the Ear

Discharge form the ear, known as otorrhoea in medical parlance, is usually caused by an infection in the middle ear.

Causes and Symptoms

The infection in the middle ear can be due to eczema, boils, or irritation caused by a plug of wax or foreign bodies like moths. This, in turn, may lead to a discharge in the external ear.

Remedies

Margosa Oil: The use of this oil has been found effective in infection and inflammation of the ear. One or two drops of this oil can be put into the ear two or three times daily with beneficial results.

Breast Milk: The use of breast milk is a popular remedy for the inflammatory condition of the ear. A few drops of this milk put into the affected ear will give relief. Mother's milk would be preferable, but if it is not available, the milk of any healthy lactating woman can be used.

Onion: Onion is beneficial for the treatment of pus in the ear. The juice extracted from an onion should be slightly warmed and put into the ear two or three times daily. It will bring good results.

Dietary Considerations

An exclusive diet of fresh juicy fruits for three to five days is advised. After that, the patient may gradually adopt a well-balanced diet, with emphasis on wholegrain cereals, raw or lightly-cooked vegetables, and fresh fruits. The patient should avoid white flour, sugar, and all products made from them; pickles, condiments, and flesh foods. Phelgm-increasing foods like milled rice, sugar, and lentils should be avoided.

Other Measures

During the initial fruit fast, a warm-water enema should be used daily to cleanse the system. Regular exercises, outdoor games, and fresh air are important. The patient should sit in the sun for fifteen minutes to allow sunlight to penetrate the inner part of his ear. This will help to stop the discharge of pus from the ear.

Eczema

The term eczema refers to an inflammation of the skin which results in the formation of vesicles or pustules. It is a common and troublesome condition of the skin. The disease has a wide variety of forms, the majority of them being of chronic variety.

Causes and Symptoms

Eczema in its acute form presents redness and swelling of the skin, and the formation of minute vesicles. If the vesicles rupture, a raw, moist surface is formed, from which a colourless discharge oozes, forming crusts on the skin where it accumulates. The symptoms are usually worse at night. The skin itches at all stages.

Eczema is essentially a constitutional disease, resulting from a toxic condition of the system, and failure of the human system to excrete the poisons from the various orifices of the body. Other causes include faulty metabolism, constipation, nutritional deficiencies, menstrual stress, jealousy, frustration, and a host of other emotions. Suppressive drug treatment of another disease is also a potent, subsidiary causative factor in many cases.

Remedies

Musk Melon: Musk melon is regarded as one of the most effective remedies for eczema. In fact, 'melon cure' can be successfully employed in the treatment of this disease. In this mode of treatment, only musk melons should be taken three times during the day for forty days or more. In the beginning, only 3 kg of melons are taken daily for three days. Then the quantity is increased by 1 kg daily till it is sufficient to appease the hunger. Only the sweet and fresh fruits of the best variety are used. As the water content of the fruit is above 90 per cent, no water should be taken during this period. The juice of the fruit is also beneficial for local application in chronic and acute cases of eczema.

Mango: Mangoes are considered another effective remedy for eczema. The pulp and the skin of the fruit should be simmered in a cup of water for half an hour. This should then be strained and applied as a lotion liberally to all affected areas several times daily.

Vegetable Juices: Raw vegetable juices, especially carrot juice in combination with spinach juice, have proved beneficial in the treatment of eczema. The formula proportions considered helpful in this combination are 300 ml of carrot juice and 200 ml of spinach juice to make 500 ml or 1/2 litre of the juice.

Finger Millet Leaves: The green leaves of finger millet are valuable in chronic eczema. The fresh juice of these leaves should be applied over the affected area in the treatment of this condition.

Safflower Oil: It has been established in laboratory animal tests that eczema can result from lack of linoleic acid. Safflower oil, being rich in this acid, can be beneficially used in the treatment of eczema. Two tablespoons of this oil should be taken daily in treating this disease. The quantity can be reduced to one tablespoon daily after the condition improves.

Blackstrap Molasses: Blackstrap molasses have been found beneficial in the treatment of this disease. This is presumably due to their high nutritive properties. Two tablespoons of molasses should be taken twice daily in a glass of milk. Improvements will be noticeable within two weeks' time.

Dietary Considerations

The treatment should start with a fast of orange juice and water for five to ten days, depending on the severity and duration of the trouble. This will help eliminate toxic waste from the body and lead to substantial improvement. Fruits, salt-free raw or steamed vegetables with wholemeal bread or *chapatis* may be taken after the juice fast. Coconut oil may be used instead of ghee. After a few days, curd and milk may be added to the diet. The patient may, thereafter, gradually embark upon a well-balanced diet, consisting of seeds, nuts, grains, vegetables, and fruits. He should avoid tea, coffee, alcoholic beverages, all condiments, sugar, white flour products, denatured cereals, and highly flavoured dishes.

Other Measures

Sunbathing is beneficial as it kills the harmful bacteria and should be resorted to early in the morning, at the first light of dawn. A light mudpack applied over the sites of the eczema is also helpful. The pack should be applied for an hour at a time and should be repeated twice or thrice a day. In cases of acute eczema, cold compress, or cold wet fomentations are beneficial. The affected part should be wrapped with thick soft cloth. The treatment for chronic eczema is just the opposite of the one for the acute problem. A hot compress or hot fomentation should be applied for twenty minutes and should be followed with a cold water bath.

Certain liquids have been found useful as washing lotions for cleaning the affected parts. These include water in which *neem* leaves have been boiled, rice starch water obtained by decanting cooked rice, and turmeric water prepared by boiling water to which turmeric powder has been added.

The patient should get as much fresh air as possible. Restrictive clothing should not be worn. Two or three litres of water should be drunk daily, and the patient must bathe twice or thrice a day. The skin, with the exception of the parts affected with eczema, should be vigorously rubbed with the palms of the hands before taking a bath.

Epilepsy

Falling Sickness

Epilepsy refers to a condition in which fits or attacks of unconsciousness occur, with or without convulsions. Known as 'falling sickness', it is a serious disorder of the central nervous system. It occurs in both children and adults. Most attacks, however, occur in childhood and in early adult life.

Causes and Symptoms

There are two main types of epilepsy known as petit mal and grand mal. In petit mal, an attack starts and stops within a few seconds. The patient has a momentary loss of consciousness, with no convulsions except sometimes a slight rigidity. The attack in the case of grand mal comes with a dramatic effect. There are violent contractions of the arms, legs, and the rest of the body, accompanied by a sudden loss of consciousness. In a typical attack, the patient cries out; falls to the ground; loses consciousness; and develops convulsions, with foaming at the mouth, twitching of the muscles, biting of the tongue, distorted fixation of limbs, rotation of the head, and deviation of the eyes.

The main cause of petit mal is a strained nervous condition.

Grand mal results from hereditary influences, serious shock or injury to the brain or nervous system, and diseases like meningitis and typhoid. Other causes of epilepsy include allergic reaction to certain food substances, circulatory disorders, chronic alcoholism, lead poisoning, use of cocaine and other such habits, mental conflict, and deficient mineral assimilation.

Remedies

Grape Juice: Fruits like apples, figs, and grapes have proved beneficial in the treatment of epilepsy. The juice of grapes has, however, been found to be comparatively more effective for this disease. The patient should take about 500 ml of the juice of fresh grapes thrice a day for three months. It will provide immense relief and help in the cure of the disease.

Vegetable Juices: Certain vegetable juices, especially carrot juice, in combination with juices of beets and cucumber, have also been found valuable in epilepsy. The formula proportions considered helpful in this combination are 300 ml of carrot juice and 100 ml each of beet and cucumber juices to prepare 500 ml or half a litre of mixed juice to be taken daily.

Vitamin B_6: Vitamin B_6 or pyridoxine is considered useful in epilepsy. This vitamin is involved in critical functions of the nervous system. The valuable vegetable sources of this vitamin are rice, milk, brewer's yeast, cereals, legumes, green leafy vegetables, carrots, and peanuts. If taken in supplement form, vitamin B_6 should be taken in therapeutic dose of 100–150 mg daily, along with other B complex vitamins.

Brahmi Booti: The herb *brahmi booti*, botanically known as *Herpesties monniera* has been found valuable in epilepsy. A teaspoon of the juice of this plant, sweetened with a teaspoon of honey, should be given to the patient thrice daily.

Indian Spikenard: The herb is also considered useful in epilepsy. It soothes the nervous system and induces tranquillity of the mind. It should be given in very small doses of one gram or so, once daily.

Valerian: The herb valerian has acquired a great reputation in recent years as a cure for epilepsy. It has been used traditionally in functional disturbances of the nervous system. The drug exercises depressant action on the central nervous system. An infusion, prepared by infusing thirty grams of the herb in half a litre of boiling water, should be taken in equal parts thrice daily.

Dietary Considerations

To begin with, the patient should be placed on an exclusive fruit diet for the first few days. During this period, he should have three meals a day of fresh juicy fruits such as oranges, apples, grapes, grapefruit, peaches, pears, pineapples, and melons. Thereafter, he may gradually adopt a well-balanced diet consisting of seeds, nuts, grains, vegetables, and fruits, with emphasis on sprouted seeds such as alfalfa seeds and moong beans, raw vegetables, and fruits. The diet should include a moderate amount of unboiled milk, preferably goat's milk, and milk products such as raw butter and home-made cottage cheese. The diet should completely eliminate all animal proteins except milk. The patient should avoid all refined foods, fried and greasy foods, sugar and products made with it, strong tea, coffee, alcoholic beverages, condiments, and pickles. He should avoid overeating and take frequent small meals rather than a few large ones.

Other Measures

Epileptics should strictly adhere to a routine with fixed timings for meals and rest. They should remain mentally active but avoid all severe mental and physical stress. Above all, they should avoid excitement of all kinds.

Fatigue

Exhaustion

Almost every one has to work long hours on certain occasions, sacrificing rest and sleep. This may cause temporary fatigue.

Causes and Symptoms

Fatigue refers to a feeling of tiredness or weariness. It can be temporary or chronic. This condition can be remedied by adequate rest. Chronic or continuous fatigue is, however, a serious problem which requires a comprehensive plan of treatment.

A specific character trait, compulsiveness, can lead to continuous fatigue. Many persons constantly feel that they cannot take rest until they finish everything that needs to be done at one time. These persons are usually tense and cannot relax unless they complete the whole job, no matter how tired they may be.

The main cause of fatigue is lowered vitality or lack of energy due to wrong feeding habits. The habitual use of refined foods such as white sugar, refined cereals, white flour products, and processed foods have very bad effect on the system in general. Foods 'denatured' in this way are deprived, to a very great extent, of their invaluable vitamins and minerals. Certain physical and mental conditions can cause fatigue. These include anaemia, intestinal worms, low blood pressure, low blood sugar, any kind of infection in the body, liver damage, allergy to foods and drugs, insomnia, mental tension, and unresolved emotional problems. Poisons and toxins resulting from air, soil, and water pollution can also lead to fatigue.

Remedies

Cereal Seeds: The patient suffering from fatigue should eat nutritious foods which supply energy to the body. Cereal seeds in their natural state relieve fatigue and provide energy. These cereal seeds are corn seeds, wheat seeds, rye seeds, maize seeds, barley seeds, and oat seeds. They must be freshly milled. In uncooked cereals we have a perfect food for perfect health which contain the essential vitamins and energy creators. In addition to cereal seeds, fresh raw nuts should be taken directly.

B Vitamins: The patient should also take natural vitamins and mineral supplements as an effective assurance against nutritional deficiencies as such deficiencies cause fatigue. Lack of pantothenic acid, a B vitamin, in particular, leads to extreme fatigue as deficiency of this vitamin is associated with exhaustion of the adrenal glands. A daily dosage of 30 mg of pantothenic acid or vitamin B_5 is recommended. However the entire B complex group should be taken, with the recommended quantity of pantothenic acid, so as to avoid imbalance of some of the other B vitamins. In fact the entire B complex group protects nerves and increases energy by helping to nourish and regulate glands. Foods rich in vitamin B are brewer's yeast, wheat germ. rice polishings, and liver.

Minerals: Minerals are also important. Potassium is essential for protection against fatigue. Green leafy vegetables, oranges, potatoes and lentils are rich in this mineral. Calcium is essential for relaxation and is beneficial in cases of insomnia and tension, both of which can lead to fatigue. Milk and milk products, green vegetables, sesame seeds, almonds, oats, and walnuts are rich sources of calcium. Sodium and zinc are also beneficial in the treatment of fatigue. Foods such as celery, cucumber, lettuce, and apples are good sources of sodium; while legumes, wholegrain products and pumpkin seeds contain ample quantities of zinc.

Dates: Dates are an effective home remedy for fatigue and those suffering from tiredness should consume them regularly. Five to seven dates should be soaked overnight in half a cup of water and crushed in the morning in the same water after removing the seeds. This water with the essence of the dates should be taken at least twice a week.

Grapefruit: Grapefruit has been found valuable in allaying fatigue. Taking a glass of grapefruit and lemon juice in equal parts is an excellent way of dispelling fatigue and general tiredness after a day's work.

Lemon Balm: The herb lemon balm is also very useful for brain fatigue or mental tiredness. A cold infusion of the balm should be taken freely in the treatment of this condition. This infusion is prepared by placing thirty grams of the herb in half a litre of cold water and allowing it to stand for twelve hours. It is then strained and taken in small doses throughout the day.

Dietary Considerations

Nutritional measures are most vital in the treatment of fatigue. Studies reveal that people who eat snacks in-between meals suffer less from fatigue and nervousness, think more clearly, and are more efficient than those who eat only three meals daily. These snacks should consist of fresh or dried fruits, fresh fruit or vegetable juices, raw vegetables, or small sandwiches of wholegrain bread. These snacks should be light and less food should be consumed at regular meals. The snacks should also be taken at specified timings such as 11 a.m., 4 p.m., and before retiring.

Other Measures

Chronic fatigue caused by poor circulation can be remedied by daily physical exercise. It will help relieve tension, bring a degree of freshness, renew energy, and induce sleep. Brisk walking, bicycling, gardening, playing tennis or golf are all good forms of exercise.

Massage, cold applications increasing in degree gradually, or alternate hot and cold baths, stimulate the muscles to renewed activity, thereby relieving fatigue. They do not simply deaden the sense of fatigue as follows the use of tea or coffee, but have a real tonic effect.

Female Sterility

Sterility in females refers to the incapacity to conceive and give birth to a living baby. Sterility or failure to reproduce must be distinguished from frigidity which denotes failure to perform the sex act or performing it imperfectly.

Causes and Symptoms

Female sterility may be due to physical defects, physical debility, and functional faults. Sterility due to physical debility can result from poor health as a consequence of certain acute or chronic diseases. Complaints like gonorrhoea, syphilis, and inflammation of the fallopian tubes also come under this category. Chronic anaemia, constipation, and leucorrhoea aggravate these conditions. Sterility may also be caused by loss of essential glands or organs of reproduction, or a decrease in their functions. Obesity or emaciation due either to dietetic errors or faulty metabolism are other factors which can contribute to female sterility. Psychological factors like emotional stress, tension, mental depression, anxiety, and fear may also result in psychosomatic sterility. This condition is generally temporary and can be corrected by psychotherapy.

Remedies

The patient should be seen by a specialist so that the specific cause is found and treated.

The following measures are helpful:

Banyan Roots: The tender roots of the banyan tree are one of the valuable remedies found beneficial in the treatment of female sterility where there are no organic defects or congenital deformities. These roots should be dried in the shade and finely powdered. About twenty grams of this powder should be mixed with milk, which should be five times the weight of the powder, and taken at night for three consecutive nights after the monthly periods are over. When this remedy is administered, no other food should be eaten for a short while thereafter. This remedy should be repeated after the completion of the menstrual cycle every month till conception takes place.

Jambul Leaves: An infusion of the fresh tender leaves of jambul fruit is an excellent remedy for sterility or miscarriage due to an ovarian or endometrium functional disorder. The infusion can be prepared by pouring 250 ml of boiling water over 20 gm of fresh jambul leaves, and allowing it to steep for two hours. The infusion may be taken with either two teaspoons of honey or 200 ml of buttermilk.

Winter Cherry: The herb winter cherry is another valuable remedy found helpful in sterility. The herb should be powdered and six grams of this powder should be taken with one cup of milk for five to six nights after menstruation.

Nutrients: Certain nutrients, especially vitamins C and E, and zinc, have been found helpful in some cases of sterility. A woman who is unable to conceive should take 1000 mg of vitamin C, 100 I.U. of vitamin E and 30 mg of zinc daily.

Dietary Considerations

Physical debility and functional faults of organic nature can be cured by simple and effective methods of natural treatment, of which optimum nutrition is an essential part. Fasting is the best remedy for the treatment of disorders resulting from toxins in the system. A short fast of two or three days should be undertaken at regular intervals by women who are unable to bear children.

Diet is an important factor in the treatment of sterility. It should contain seeds, nuts, grains, vegetables, and fruits. These foods should be supplemented with milk, vegetable oils, and honey. Curd and cottage cheese are also recommended. About seventy to eighty per cent of the diet should consist of foods in their natural uncooked state, because cooking destroys much of the nutritional value of most foods. Sprouting is an excellent way of consuming seeds, beans, and grains in their raw form, as in the process of sprouting, the nutritional value is multiplied, new vitamins are created and the protein quality is improved. Excessive fat, spicy foods, strong tea, coffee, white sugar, white flour, refined cereals, flesh foods, greasy or fried foods should all be avoided.

Other Measures

The bowels should be cleansed by a warm-water enema during the period of fasting and afterwards when necessary. This will have a beneficial effect not only on the digestive system but also on the surrounding organs of the urinary and genital system. Other helpful measures in overcoming female sterility are mud packs and cold water treatments like a hip bath and wet girdle pack. These treatments greatly improve internal circulation in the genital organs and relieve them of all kinds of inflammation and other abnormalities. Mud packs may be applied to the abdomen and sexual organs. The cold hip bath should be taken for ten minutes at a water temperature of $10^0C-18.3^0C$. For a wet girdle pack, a thin underwear wrung in cold water should be worn. Over this, a thick, dry cotton or woollen underwear should be worn. All cold treatments should be suspended during menstruation.

Certain *yogasanas* which are said to tone up the gonads or ovaries should also be practised regularly for overcoming female sterility. These *asanas* are *sarvangasana*, *matsyasana*, *ardhamatsyendrasana*, *paschimottanasana* and *shalabhasana*.

All these measures, along with clean habits, proper rest, and relaxation will go a long way in overcoming female sterility.

Gall-Bladder Disorders

Inflammation of Gall-Bladder, Gallstones

The main problems which afflict the gall-bladder are an inflammatory condition known as cholecystitis and the presence of gallstones in the gall-bladder. The latter condition is called cholelithiasis. The former often leads to the latter. Gallstones are usually caused by disturbances in the composition of the bile.

Causes and Symptoms

The main symptom of gall-bladder disease is acute or inter-mittent pain in the abdomen. Indigestion, gas, a feeling of fullness after meals, constipation, and nausea are the other usual symptoms. Intolerance to fats, dizziness, jaundice, anaemia, acne, and other lesions may also occur.

The main cause of gall-bladder disorders is overnutrition resulting from excessive intake of refined carbohydrates, especially sugar. Overnutrition also leads to increased cholesterol secretion.

Meals rich in fats may cause an attack of gall-bladder pain or gallstone colic. Other causes are chronic constipation, poor health, hereditary factors, and stress. The Chinese relate gall-bladder disorders with the emotion of anger.

Remedies

Beet: The fresh juice of beets, and the juices of carrot and cucumber in quantities of 100 ml each, are one of the finest cleansers of the gall-bladder. This combined juice has proved beneficial in the treatment of all disorders related to this organ, and should be taken twice daily.

Pear: The pear is another excellent remedy for gall-bladder disorders. The fruit or its juice should be taken liberally by the patient with beneficial results. It exercises a special healing effect on all gall-bladder disorders, including gallstones.

Chicory: The flowers, seeds, and roots of chicory or the endive plant are considered valuable in gall-bladder disorders. A decoction of about 30—60 ml of the flowers, seeds, or roots can be used three times daily with beneficial results in the treatment of these disorders. Endive or chicory juice in almost any combination promotes the secretion of bile and is, therefore, very good for both liver and gall-bladder dysfunctions.

Dandelion: Dandelion has a beneficial effect on the gall-bladder. About 125 ml each of the juices of dandelion and water cress should be taken twice daily. Combined with a vegetarian diet, without much sugar and starch, these juices help to make the gall-bladder normal.

Olive and Sunflower Oil: An oil cure has been advocated by some nature cure practitioners for the removal of gallstones. Raw, natural, unrefined vegetable oils of olive or sunflower are used. The procedure is to take 30 ml of vegetable oil, preferably olive oil, first thing in the morning and follow it immediately with 120 ml of grapefruit juice or lemon juice. This treatment should be taken every morning for several days, even weeks, if necessary.

Dietary Considerations

Smaller gallstones can usually be cleared through dietetic cure. In cases of acute gall-bladder inflammation, the patient should fast for two or three days until the acute condition is cleared. Nothing but water should be taken during this period. After the fast, the patient should take fruit and vegetable juices for a few days

Carrots, beets, grapefruit, pears, lemons or grapes may be taken in the form of juice. Thereafter, the patient should adopt a well-balanced diet, with emphasis on raw and cooked vegetables, fruit and vegetable juices, and a moderate amount of fruits and seeds. Yoghurt, cottage cheese, and a tablespoon of olive oil twice a day should also be included in the diet. The patient should avoid meat, eggs, animal fats, processed and denatured foods, fried and greasy foods, refined carbohydrates, alcohol, products made with sugar and coffee, as well as spices, condiments, and pickles. The patient should eat frequent small meals rather than three large meals.

Other Measures

The pain of gallstone colic can be relieved by the application of hot packs or fomentation to the upper abdominal area. A warm-water enema at body temperature will help eliminate faecal accumulations if the patient is constipated. Physical exercise is also essential. Surgery becomes necessary if the gallstones are very large or in cases where they have been present for long.

Gastritis

Inflammation of the Stomach

Gastritis is an inflammation of the lining of the stomach. The inflammatory lesions may be either acute or chronic.

Causes and Symptoms

The main symptoms of gastritis are loss of appetite, nausea, vomiting, headache, and dizziness. There is pain and discomfort in the region of the stomach. Other symptoms are a coated tongue, foul breath, bad taste in the mouth, increased flow of saliva, scanty urination, a general feeling of uneasiness, and mental depression. In more chronic cases, the patient complaints of heartburn and a feeling of fullness in the abdomen, especially after meals. Often there is constipation, but occasionally, there may be diarrhoea due to intestinal catarrh.

The most frequent cause of gastritis is a dietetic indiscretion such as habitual overeating; eating of badly combined or improperly cooked foods; excessive intake of strong tea, coffee, or alcoholic drinks; or habitual use of large quantities of condiments and sauces. Other causes include worry, anxiety, grief, prolonged tension, use of certain drugs, strong acids, and caustic substances.

Remedies

Coconut: Coconut water is an excellent remedy for gastritis. It gives the stomach the necessary rest and provides vitamins and minerals. The stomach is greatly helped in returning to a normal condition if nothing but coconut water is given during the first twenty-four hours.

Rice: Rice gruel is another excellent remedy for acute cases of gastritis. One cup of rice gruel is recommended twice daily. In chronic cases where the flow of gastric juice is meagre, such foods as require prolonged vigorous mastication are beneficial as they induce a greater flow of gastric juice.

Potato: Potato juice has been found valuable in relieving gastritis. The recommended dose is half a cup of the juice, two or three times daily, half an hour before meals.

Marigold: The herb marigold is also considered beneficial in the treatment of gastritis. An infusion of the herb in doses of a tablespoon may be taken twice daily.

Dietary Considerations

The patient should undertake a fast for two or three days or more, depending on the severity of the condition. He should be given only warm water to drink during this period. This will give rest to the stomach and allow the toxic condition causing the inflammation to subside. After the acute symptoms subside, the patient should adopt an all-fruit diet for the next three days and take juicy fruits such as apples, pears, grapes, grapefruit, oranges, pineapple, peaches, and melons. He may, thereafter, gradually embark upon a balanced diet consisting of seeds, nuts, grains, vegetables, and fruits.

The patient should avoid the use of alcohol, tobacco, spices and condiments, meat, red pepper, sour foods, pickles, strong tea and coffee. He should also avoid sweets, pastries, rich cakes, and aerated waters. Curds and cottage cheese should be used freely. Too many different foods should not be mixed at the same meal. Meals should be taken at least two hours before going to bed at night. Eight to ten glasses of water should be taken daily but water should not be taken with meals as it dilutes the digestive juices and delays digestion. Above all, haste should be avoided while eating and meals should be served in a pleasing and relaxed atmosphere.

Other Measures

From the commencement of the treatment, a warm-water enema should be used daily for about a week to cleanse the bowels. The patient should be given dry friction and a sponge daily. Application of heat with a hot compress or hot water bottle, twice a day, either on an empty stomach or two hours after meals, will also be beneficial. The patient should not undertake any hard physical and mental work. He should, however, undertake breathing and other light exercises like walking, swimming, and golf. He should avoid worries and mental tension.

Goitre

Swelling in the Neck

Goitre refers to a swelling of the thyroid gland in the neck. Women are more prone to this disease than men.

Causes and Symptoms

The initial symptoms of goitre may be emotional upsets which gradually increase in duration. Other symptoms which appear subsequently are loss of power of concentration, irritability, and depression. The thyroid gland may swell but this has no relation to the severity of the ailment.

Deficiency of iodine in the diet is the most common cause of goitre. The thyroid gland makes use of organic iodine in its secretion and a diet deficient in organic iodine is a predisposing factor towards the appearance of this disease, especially under physical and emotional disturbances. Goitre gradually affects those who habitually live on denatured foods and not those who eat much of their food in a raw or uncooked state.

Remedies

Iodine: Iodine is, undoubtedly, most helpful in many cases, but it should be given in its organic form. All foods containing iodine should be taken liberally. These are lettuce, turnips, carrots, garlic, onions, oats, pineapples, whole rice, tomatoes, watercress, strawberries, guavas, citrus fruits, egg yolks, and sea foods.

Watercress: Watercress is one of the best sources of the element iodine. It is valuable in correcting the functioning of the thyroid gland. Its regular use, therefore, is highly beneficial in the prevention and treatment of goitre. A paste made of this vegetable can also be applied beneficially over the affected parts. It helps to reduce swelling.

Swamp Cabbage: The leaves of swamp cabbage are useful in expothalmic goitre. A teaspoon of the juice with tea almonds should be given once or twice daily as a medicine. The leaves are also useful in myxodema, a condition that results from lack of thyroid hormones.

Kachnar: *Kachnar,* botanically known as *Bauhinia variegata,* has been used as a folk medicine for goitre in India. About 30 ml of the decoction of the bark should be given twice a day in the morning on an empty stomach.

Dandelion: Dandelion has been found valuable in goitre. The leaves of this salad vegetable should be smeared with ghee, warmed and bandaged over the swollen parts for about two weeks. Any existing discomfort will be relieved by this remedy.

Flex: The seeds of flex are also useful in reducing swellings in goitre. The seeds should be ground in water, heated and applied over the affected parts. The leaves of the tree should then be bandaged over them.

Dietary Considerations

To begin with, the patient should take juices of fruits such as oranges, apples, pineapples, and grapes every two or three hours for five days. After the juice fast, the patient may spend the next three days on fruits and milk, taking three meals a day of juicy fruits with a glass of milk, at five-hourly intervals. Certain foods and fluids are extremely injurious for goitre patients and should be avoided by them. These include white flour products, white sugar, flesh foods, fried or greasy foods, preserves, condiments, tea, coffee, and alcohol.

Other Measures

For the first five days of the treatment the bowels should be cleansed daily with lukewarm water. The patient should take plenty of rest and spend a day in bed every week for the first two months of the treatment. More and more physical exercise should be taken after the symptoms subside.

Gout

Painful Bony Joint

Gout refers to a certain form of inflammation of the joints and swellings of a recurrent type. Although chronic in character, it occurs in acute attacks. It is a disease of the wealthy and chiefly affects middle-aged men. Women, after menopause, are also sometimes affected by this disease.

Causes and Symptoms

An attack of gout is usually accompanied by acute pain in the big toe, which becomes tender, hot, and swollen in a few hours. It may also similarly affect other joints such as the knees and wrists, and sometimes more than one joint may be affected at a time. The attack usually occurs at midnight or in the early hours of the morning when the patient is suddenly awakened. The acute attack generally lasts for a week or so. During this period, the patient may run a slight fever, and feel disinclined to eat. A serious complication of gout is the presence of kidney stones containing uric acid. In some cases the kidneys become damaged and do not function properly.

The chief cause of gout is the formation of uric acid crystals in the joints, skin, and kidneys. Uric acid is an end product of the body's chemical processes. Those affected by gout have a higher level of uric acid in the blood than the normal, due either to formation of increased amounts or reduced amounts of acid being passed out by the kidneys in the urine. This uric acid usually remains dissolved in the blood. But when the blood becomes too full of it, the uric acid forms needle-shaped crystals in the joints which bring about attacks of gout. Other causes of this disease are heredity, alcoholic drinks, regular eating of foods rich in protein and carbohydrate, lack of proper exercise, and stress.

Remedies

Cherry: The cherry, sweet or sour, is considered an effective remedy for gout. This was discovered by Dr Ludwig W. Blan some forty years ago. Himself a gout sufferer, Blan found the use of cherries to be miraculously effective in his own case, and he published his own experience in a medical journal. Subsequently many people with gout used this simple therapy with great success. To start with, the patient should consume about fifteen to twenty five cherries a day. Thereafter, about ten cherries a day will keep the ailment under control. While fresh cherries are best, canned cherries can also be used with success.[1]

Vegetable Juices: Raw vegetable juices are protective against gout. Carrot juice, in combination with the juices of beet and cucumber, is especially valuable. Beet juice — 100 ml and cucumber juice — 100 ml should be mixed with 300 ml of carrot juice to make 500 ml of combined juice and taken daily.

French Beans: The juice of French or string beans has also proved effective in the treatment of gout. About 150 ml of this juice should be taken daily by the patient suffering from this disease.

Apple: Apples are regarded as an excellent medicine for gout. The malic acid contained in them is believed to neutralise the uric acid and afford relief to the sufferers. The patient is advised to take one apple after each meal.

Banana: Bananas have been found beneficial in the treatment of gout. A diet of bananas only for three or four days is advised. A patient can take eight or nine bananas daily during this period and nothing else.

Lime: Lime is also used as a remedy in gout. vitamin C is known to prevent and cure sore joints by strengthening the connective tissues of the body. The citric acid found in lime is a solvent of the uric acid which is the primary cause of this disease. The juice of half a lime, squeezed into a glass of water, should be taken twice daily.

Dietary Considerations

For an acute attack, there is no better remedy than a fast of orange juice and water. In severe cases, it is advisable to undertake a series of short fasts for three days or so rather than one long fast.

---

1. Quoted in Mark Bricklin's *Natural Home Remedies*, Rodale Press, India, 1986.

After the acute symptoms subside, the patient may adopt an all-fruit diet for another three or four days. Thereafter, he may gradually embark upon a well-balanced diet of natural foods, with emphasis on fresh fruits, raw vegetables, and sprouts. The patient should avoid all purine and uric acid-producing foods such as all meats, eggs, and fish; tea, coffee, sugar, white flour and its products; and all canned, processed, and fried foods.

Other Measures

A warm-water enema should be used daily during the period of fasting to cleanse the bowels. Epsom salts foot baths are advised twice daily. About 250 gm – 500gm of these salts may be added to tolerably hot water for this purpose. Full Epsom salts baths should also be taken three times a week. The baths may be reduced to two per week later. Cold packs, applied to the affected joints at night, will be beneficial. Fresh air and outdoor exercise are also essential. The patient should eliminate as much stress from his life as possible.

Halitosis

Bad Breath

Halitosis refers to foul or bad breath, which is not an uncommon condition. Unfortunately, most people who offend in this respect are completely unaware of their problem.

Causes and Symptoms

The most common cause of halitosis is diseased gums. Dental decay at the roots of the teeth may result in abscesses in the gums with foul-smelling pus, giving an objectionable odour to the breath. Even small holes in the teeth may provide a place where germs can multiply and release foul odours.

Other causes of halitosis are any conditions of the nose, throat, respiratory tract, or stomach which are associated with chronic infection or local upsets of one sort or another, such as chronic tonsillitis, lung diseases like chronic bronchitis and bronchiectasis, chronic gastritis, and sinusitis which causes a discharge at the back of the throat. Many cases of bad breath, however, are caused by gastro-intestinal disorders, intestinal sluggishness and particularly by chronic constipation.

Remedies

Fenugreek: Among the several home remedies for halitosis, the use of fenugreek has proved most effective. A tea made from the seeds of this vegetable should be taken regularly for correcting the condition. This tea is prepared by putting one teaspoon of seeds in half a litre of cold water and allowing it to simmer for fifteen minutes over a low flame. It should then be strained and used as tea.

Avocado: Another effective remedy for bad breath is avocado which is far superior to any mouth lotion or remedies for this condition. It effectively removes intestinal putrefaction or decomposition which is one of the most important causes of bad breath.

Guava: Unripe guava is useful in halitosis. It is rich in tannic, malic, oxalic, and phosphoric acids as well as calcium, oxalate, and manganese. Chewing it is an excellent tonic for the teeth and gums. It helps cure bleeding from gums and stops bad breath. Chewing tender leaves of guava tree also stops bleeding from gums and bad breath.

Parsley: Parsley is a valuable cure for bad breath. Two cups of water should be boiled and several sprigs of parsley, coarsely chopped, should be steeped in this water along with two or three whole cloves or a quarter teaspoon of ground cloves. This mixture should be stirred occasionally while cooling. It should then be strained and used as a mouthwash or gargle several times a day.

Raw Juices: All fruit and vegetable juices are beneficial in the treatment of halitosis and should be taken liberally by those suffering from this disorder. Juices from green vegetables are especially valuable.

Dietary Considerations

Patients suffering from halitosis should take a well-balanced diet consisting of seeds, nuts, grains, vegetables, and fruits, with emphasis on raw and cooked vegetables, and fruits. In case of constipation, all measures should be adopted for its eradication. The patient should avoid refined carbohydrate foods, such as white sugar, white bread and products made from them, as well as meat and eggs.

Other Measures

The teeth should be cleaned twice a day, especially before going to bed at night. Meat particles should be removed carefully with toothpicks. In case of decaying teeth and swollen and bleeding gums, a dentist should be consulted. Munching a raw apple or guava after lunch removes most of the trapped particles. The use of the twigs of the margosa *(neem)* tree as a toothbrush is the best method of cleaning the teeth.

Headache

Common Headache

Headaches afflict almost everyone at some time or the other. Most headaches are functional, being caused by temporary upsets, and are not related to any organic changes in the brain. They are often nature's warning that something is wrong somewhere in the body. The actual pain, however, arises from irritation to nerve endings in the shoulder, neck, and scalp muscles, and also in the smooth muscles encircling the blood vessels which serve these areas.

Causes and Symptoms

The common causes of headaches are allergy, emotional stress, eye strain, high blood pressure, a hangover, infection, low blood sugar, nutritional deficiency, tension, and the presence of poisons and toxins in the body. Allergies are often the unsuspected cause of headaches. The foods to which some people are allergic and which can trigger headaches are milk and milk products, chocolates, chicken, liver, alcohol, and strong cheese. Sneezing and diarrhoea are further indications of an allergy.

Remedies

Lemon: There are several remedies for various types of headaches. Lemon is beneficial in its treatment. The juice of three or four slices of lemon should be squeezed in a cup of tea and taken by the patient for treating this condition. It gives immediate relief. The crust of lemon, which is generally thrown away, has been found useful in headaches caused by heat. Lemon crusts should be pounded into a fine paste in a mortar and applied as plaster on the forehead. Applying the yellow, freshly pared-off rind of a lemon to each temple will also give relief.

Apple: Apples are valuable in all types of headaches. After removing the upper rind and the inner hard portion of a ripe apple, it should be taken with a little salt every morning on an empty stomach in such cases. This should be continued for about a week.

Henna: The flowers of henna have been found valuable in headaches caused by hot sun. The flowers should be rubbed in vinegar and applied over the forehead. This remedy will soon provide relief.

Cinnamon: Cinnamon is useful in headaches caused by exposure to cold air. A fine paste of this spice should be prepared by mixing it with water and it should be applied over the temples and forehead to obtain relief.

Marjoram: The herb marjoram is beneficial in the treatment of a nervous headache. An infusion of the leaves is taken as a tea in the treatment of this disorder.

Rosemary: The herb rosemary has been found valuable in headaches resulting from cold. A handful of this herb should be boiled in a litre of water and put in a mug. The head should be covered with a towel and the steam inhaled for as long as the patient can bear. This should be repeated till the headache is relieved.

Dietary Considerations

The best way to prevent headaches is to build up physical resistance through proper nutrition, physical exercise and positive thinking. As a first step, the patient should undertake a short fast, and take citrus fruit juices diluted with water every two hours from 8.00 a.m. to 8.00 p.m. daily. Thereafter, he should plan his diet in such a way as to put the least possible strain on the digestion. Breakfast may consist of fruits, both fresh and dried. Lunch may consist of protein foods. Starchy foods such as wholewheat bread, cereals, rice, or potatoes should be taken at dinner along with raw salads. Spices, condiments, sour buttermilk, and oily foodstuffs should be avoided. Drinking a glass of water (warm water in winter and cool water in summer), mixed with a teaspoon of honey first thing in the morning, is also a good remedy. Copious drinking of water throughout the day is also advised.

Other Measures

Other helpful measures in the treatment of headaches are a cleansing enema with water temperature at 37⁰C, a cold throat pack, frequent applications of towels wrung out from very hot water to the back of the neck, a cold compress at 4.4⁰C to 15.6⁰C applied to the head and face, or an alternate spinal compress. Hot fomentations over the abdominal region just before retiring relieve headaches caused by stomach and liver upsets.

Hot foot baths are also beneficial in the treatment of chronic headaches. The patient should keep his legs in a tub or bucket filled with hot water at a temperature of 40⁰C to 45⁰C for fifteen minutes every night before retiring. This treatment should be continued for two or three weeks.

Yogic *kriyas* like *jalneti* and *kunjal*; *pranayamas* like *anuloma-viloma, shitali,* and *sitkari;* and *asanas* such as *uttanpadasana, sarvangasana, paschimottanasana, halasana,* and *shavasana* are also beneficial in the treatment of headaches.

High Blood Cholesterol

Hypercholesterolaemia

Cholesterol, a yellowish fatty substance, is one of the essential ingredients of the body. Although it is essential to life, it has a bad reputation, being a major villain in heart disease. Every person with high blood cholesterol is regarded as a potential candidate for heart attack or a stroke. Most of the cholesterol found in the body is produced in the liver. However, about twenty to thirty per cent generally comes from the foods we eat.

Cholesterol is measured in milligrams per 100 millimetres of blood. The normal level of cholesterol varies between 150 − 200 mg per 100 ml. In blood, cholesterol occurs in combination with certain lipids (fats), hence, known as lipoproteins. There are two main types of lipoproteins: a low density one (LDL) and a high density one (HDL). The low density lipoprotein is the one which is considered harmful and is associated with cholesterol deposits in blood vessels. The higher the ratio of LDL to the total cholesterol, the greater will be the risk of arterial damage and heart disease.

HDL, on the other hand, plays a salutory role by helping remove cholesterol from circulation and thereby reducing the risk of heart disease.

Causes and Symptoms

Hypercholesterolaemia or increase in cholesterol is mainly a hereditary disorder. It is also caused by taking rich foods and fried foods; excessive consumption of milk and its products like ghee, butter, and cream; white flour, sugar, cakes, pastries, biscuits, cheese, and ice cream; and non-vegetarian foods like meat, fish, and eggs. Other causes of increase in cholesterol are irregularity in habits, smoking, and drinking alcohol. Stress has also been found to be a major cause of increased level of cholesterol.

Remedies

Lecithin: Lecithin, also a fatty food substance and the most abundant of the phospholipids, is beneficial in case of increase in cholesterol level. It has the ability to break up cholesterol into small particles which can be easily handled by the system. With sufficient intake of lecithin, cholesterol cannot build up against the walls of the arteries and veins. Lecithin also increases the production of bile acids made from cholesterol, thereby reducing its amount in the blood. Egg yolk, vegetable oils, wholegrain cereals, soyabeans, and unpasturised milk are rich sources of lecithin. The cells of the body are also capable of synthesizing it as needed, if several of the B vitamins are present.

Vitamins: Vitamins B_6, choline, and inositol are particularly effective in reducing the level of blood cholesterol. Wheat germ, yeast, or vitamin B extracted from bran contain high quantities of these vitamins. Vitamin E also elevates blood lecithin and reduces cholesterol.

The patient should take liberal quantities of vitamin E - rich foods such as sunflower seeds, safflower, soyabean oils, butter, and sprouted seeds and grains.

Sunflower Seeds: Sunflower seeds are valuable in lowering high blood cholesterol. They contain a substantial quantity of linoleic acid which is the fat helpful in reducing cholesterol deposits on the walls of arteries. Substituting sunflower seeds for some of the solid fats like butter and cream will, therefore, lead to great improvement in health.

Coriander Seeds: Regular drinking of a decoction of coriander seeds helps lower blood cholesterol. It is a good diuretic and helps stimulate the kidneys. It is prepared by boiling two tablespoons of dry seeds in a glass of water, and straining the decoction after cooling. This decoction should be taken twice daily.

Ishabgul: The herb ishabgul has been found beneficial in the treatment of high cholesterol level. The oil of the seeds of this plant should be given for lowering blood cholesterol. It contains fifty per cent linoleic acid. This oil is more active than safflower oil, and one teaspoon should be taken twice daily.

Fibre: The amount of fibre in the diet also influences the cholesterol levels and LDL cholesterol can be lowered by taking diets rich in fibres. The most significant sources of dietary fibre are unprocessed wheat bran, whole cereals such as wheat, rice, barley, rye; legumes such as potatoes, carrots, beet, and turnips; fruits such as mangoes and guavas; and leafy vegetables such as cabbage, lady's fingers, lettuce, and celery. Oat bran and corn bran are specially beneficial in lowering LDL cholesterol.

Dietary Considerations

To reduce the risk of heart disease, it is essential to lower the level of LDL and increase the level of HDL. This can be achieved by a change in diet and lifestyle. As a first step, foods rich in cholesterol and saturated fats, which lead to an increase in the LDL level, should be reduced to the minimum. These foods are eggs, organic meats, cheese, butter, bacon, beef, and whole milk. Virtually all foods of animal origin, as well as two vegetable oils, namely, coconut and palm, are high in saturated fats, and these should be replaced by polyunsaturated fats such as corn, safflower, soyabean, and sesame oils which tend to lower the level of LDL.

Persons with high blood cholesterol level should drink at least eight to ten glasses of water every day, as copious drinking of water stimulates the excretory activity of the skin and kidneys. This, in turn, facilitates elimination of excessive cholesterol from the system.

Other Measures

Regular physical exercise also plays an important role in lowering LDL cholesterol and in raising the level of protective HDL. It also promotes circulation and helps maintain the blood flow to every part of the body. Jogging or brisk walking, swimming, bicycling, and playing badminton are excellent forms of exercise.

High Blood Pressure

Hypertension or high blood pressure, as it is more commonly known, is regarded as a silent killer. It is a disease of the modern age. The fast pace of life and the mental and physical pressures caused by the increasingly industrialised and metropolitan environments have a role to play in the rise in blood pressure.

Blood pressure is measured with an instrument called sphygnomanometer in millimetres of mercury. The highest pressure reached during each heart beat is called systolic pressure, and the lowest between two beats is known as diastolic pressure. Most young adults have blood pressure around 120/80. It increases normally with age, even going upto 160/90.

Causes and Symptoms

The first symptom of hypertension may appear as a pain at the back of the head and neck on waking in the morning, which soon disappears. Some of the other common symptoms are dizziness, palpitations, pain in the region of the heart, frequent urination, nervous tension, fatigue, and difficulty in breathing.

The chief causes of high blood pressure are stress and a faulty style of living. Smoking and an excessive intake of intoxicants, tea, coffee, and refined foods destroy the natural pace of life and prevent the expulsion of waste and poisonous matter from the body. Hardening of the arteries (atherosclerosis), obesity, and diabetes lead to hypertension. Other causes of high blood pressure are an excessive intake of common table salt, and eating a high fat and low fibre diet.

Remedies

Garlic: Garlic is regarded as an effective means of lowering blood pressure. It is said to reduce spasms of the small arteries. It also slows down the pulse rate and modifies the heart rhythm, besides relieving the symptoms of dizziness, numbness, shortness of breath, and the formation of gas within the digestive tract. It may be taken in the form of raw cloves or two to three capsules a day.

Indian Gooseberry: Indian gooseberry is another effective remedy for high blood pressure. A tablespoon each of fresh *amla* juice and honey mixed together should be taken every morning in this condition.

Lemon: Lemon is also regarded as a valuable food to control high blood pressure. It is a rich source of vitamin P which is found both in the juice and peel of the fruit. This vitamin is essential for preventing capillary fragility.

Grapefruit: Grapefruit is useful in preventing high blood pressure. The vitamin P content in the fruit is helpful in toning up the arteries.

Watermelon: Watermelon is another valuable safeguard against high blood pressure. A substance extracted from watermelon seeds is said to have a definite action in dilating the blood vessels, which results in lowering the blood pressure. The seeds, dried and roasted, should be taken in liberal quantities.

Rice: Rice has a low-fat, low-cholesterol, and low-salt content. It makes a perfect diet for those hypertensive persons who have been advised salt-restricted diets. Calcium in brown rice, in particular, soothes and relaxes the nervous system and helps relieve the symptoms of high blood pressure.

Potato: Potatoes, specially in boiled form, are a valuable food for lowering blood pressure. When boiled with their skin, they absorb very little salt. Thus they can form a useful addition to a salt-free diet recommended for patients with high blood pressure. Potatoes are rich in potassium but not in sodium salts. The magnesium present in the vegetable exercises beneficial effects in lowering blood pressure.

Parsley: Parsley is very useful in high blood pressure. It contains elements which help maintain the blood vessels, particularly, the capillaries. It keeps the arterial system in a healthy condition. It may be taken as a beverage by simmering 20 gm of fresh parsley leaves gently in 250 ml of water for a few minutes. This may be drunk several times daily.

Rauwolfia: Among the herbs, rauwolfia is the best remedy for high blood pressure. Alkaloids of this drug, which have a direct effect on hypertension, have been isolated and are being widely used by practitioners of modern medicine, but they have certain unpleasant side-effects which the drug, taken in raw form, does not have. Practitioners of the Indian system of medicine have, therefore, preferred to use the root of the drug in a powdered form. Half a teaspoon of this drug, taken thrice a day, is very effective in hypertension.

Vegetable Juices: Raw vegetable juices, especially carrot and spinach juices, taken separately or in combination, are also beneficial in the treatment of high blood pressure. If taken in combination, 300 ml of carrot juice and 200 ml of spinach juice should be mixed to make 500 ml or half a litre of the juice, and taken daily. If taken separately, one glass should be taken twice daily, morning and evening.

Dietary Calcium and Potassium: Recent studies have revealed an important link between dietary calcium and potassium and hypertension. Researchers have found that people who take potassium-rich diets have a low incidence of hypertension even if they do not control their salt intake. They have also found that people with hypertension do not seem to get much calcium in the form of dairy products. These two essential nutrients seem to help the body secrete excess sodium and are involved in important functions which control the working of the vascular system. Potassium is found in abundance in fruits and vegetables, and calcium in dairy products.

Dietary Considerations

Persons with high blood pressure should always follow a well-balanced routine of a proper diet, exercise, and rest. Diet is of primary importance. Meat and eggs, more than any other food, cause the blood pressure to rise. The pressure can be lowered and blood clotting diminished by increasing the consumption of fruits, reducing protein intake, and sticking to a vegetarian diet. A natural diet consisting of fresh fruits and vegetables instead of a traditional diet, helps to get rid of the toxins from the body. Salt should be avoided; in any case, it should not exceed more than three grams or about half a teaspoon per day.

Other Measures

Persons suffering from hypertension must get at least eight hours of good sleep, because proper rest is a vital aspect of the treatment. Most important of all, the patient must avoid overstrain, worries, tension, anger, and haste. He or she must develop a calm and cheerful attitude and develop a contented frame of mind.

Hysteria

Hysteria is a mental disorder arising from intense anxiety. It is characterised by lack of control over acts and emotions, and by sudden seizures of unconsciousness with emotional outbursts. It is often the result of repressed conflicts within the person. This disease appears in both sexes, but it is far more common in young women between fourteen and twenty five years of age.

Causes and Symptoms

The symptoms of hysteria are heaviness in the limbs, severe cramps, a strong feeling of ascending abdominal constriction, continual sighings, difficulty in breathing, constriction in the chest, palpitations, feeling of a foreign body lodged in the throat, swelling of the neck and of the jugular veins, suffocation, headache, clenched teeth, and generalized and voluntary tensing of muscles of locomotion. In severe cases, additional symptoms are noticeable; these may include wild and painful cries, incomplete loss of consciousness, an enormously swollen neck, violent and tumultuous heartbeats, involuntary locomotor muscle contraction, frightening generalized convulsions, and violent movement.

The physical symptoms include a weakness of the will, a craving for love and sympathy, and a tendency towards emotional instability. Hysterical trances may last for days or weeks. A patient in a trance may appear to be in a deep sleep, but the muscles are not usually relaxed.

The most common causes of hysteria are sexual repression, perverted habits of thought, and idleness. Heredity plays an important part in its causation. A nervous family background and faulty emotional training when young are predisposing causes. The emotional situations may be caused by mental strain, stress, fear, worry, depression, traumatism, masturbation, and prolonged sickness.

Remedies

Jambul: The jambul fruit is considered an effective home remedy for hysteria. Three kilograms of this fruit and a handful of salt should be put in a jug filled with water. The jug should be kept in the sun for a week. A women suffering from hysteria should take 300 gm of these fruits on an empty stomach, and drink a cup of water from the jug. The day she starts this treatment, 3 kg more of these fruits, mixed with a handful of salt, should be put in another jug filled with water, so that when the contents of the first jug are finished, the contents of the other will be ready for use. This treatment should be continued for two weeks.

Honey: Honey is regarded as another effective remedy for hysteria. It is advisable to take one tablespoon of honey daily.

Bottle Gourd: Bottle gourd is useful as an external application in hysteria. Macerated fresh pulp of this vegetable should be applied over the head of the patient in the treatment of this disease.

Lettuce: Lettuce is considered valuable in this disease. A cup of fresh juice of lettuce, mixed with a teaspoon of Indian gooseberry *(amla)* juice, should be given every day in the morning for a month, as a medicine in the treatment of hysteria.

Rauwolfia: The herb rauwolfia is very useful in hysteria. One gram of the powdered root should be administered with one cup of milk in the morning as well as in the evening. Treatment should be continued till a complete cure has been obtained.

Asafoetida: Asafoetida has also proved beneficial in the treatment of this disease. Smelling this gum prevents hysterical attacks. If taken orally, the daily dosage should be from 0.5 to 1.0 gm. An emulsion made up of 2 gm of the gum with 120 ml of water is a valuable enema in hysteria, when the patient resists taking the gum orally.

Dietary Considerations

In most cases of hysteria, it is desirable for patients to start the treatment by adopting an all-fruit diet for several days, taking three meals a day of juicy fruits such as oranges, apples, grapes, grapefruit, papayas, and pineapples. This may be followed by an exclusive milk diet for about a month. The milk diet will help to build better blood and nourish the nerves. If the full milk diet is not convenient, a diet of milk and fruits may be adopted. The patient may, thereafter, gradually embark upon a well-balanced diet of seeds, nuts, grains, vegetables, and fruits. The patient should avoid alcohol, tea, coffee, tobacco, white sugar and white flour, and products made from them.

Other Measures

The patient should be taught self-control and educated in the right habits of thinking. Her mind must be drawn away from herself by some means. Proper sex education should be provided and a married patient should be taught to enjoy a normal sexual relationship. Exercise and outdoor games are also important. They take the mind away from self and induce cheerfulness. *Yogasanas* which are useful in hysteria are *bhujangasana, shalabhasana, matsyasana, sarvangasana, dhanurasana, halasana, paschimottanasana, yogamudra,* and *shavasana.* Weak patients, who are not able to do much active exercise, may be given a massage three or four times a week.

Influenza

Flu

Influenza, also known as flu, is the clinical condition that results from infection with influenza viruses. The main effects of the influenza viruses are on the upper respiratory tract, the nose and throat, with possible spread and involvement of the lungs and bronchi. The disease is highly contagious and it has the potential to cause a widespread epidemic, affecting a sizeable portion of a population at any time.

Causes and Symptoms

Influenza strikes suddenly. It usually begins with chills, fever, headache, and severe muscular pains. The patient feels miserable and weak. There is an inflammation in the nose and throat, which may spread down the windpipe to the lungs, resulting in a sore throat, cough, and running of the nose and eyes. In milder cases, the temperature rises to 39^0C or 102^0F, and in severe cases, it may go upto 40^0C or 104^0F. The consequent weakness and fatigue may continue for several weeks.

Influenza is a viral disease. It generally affects those with a toxic and run-down condition. Such a state is brought about by dietetic errors and a faulty style of living such as worry, overwork, lack of proper exercise, living in stuffy rooms, and keeping late hours. No disease germs can find lodgement and become active in the system of a person who is perfectly healthy in the true sense of the term. Influenza is passed on with ease from the affected person to many others who are also in an equally low vital state.

Remedies

Long Pepper: The use of long pepper is one of the most effective remedies in the treatment of influenza. Half a teaspoon of the powder of long pepper, mixed with two teaspoons of honey and half a teaspoon of juice of ginger, should be taken thrice a day. This will help greatly if taken in the initial stages of the disease. It is especially useful in avoiding complications which follow the onset of the disease, namely, the involvement of the larynx and the bronchial tube.

Garlic: Garlic is an excellent remedy for influenza. It is useful as a general antiseptic and the patient should take as much as he can bear.

Turmeric: Turmeric is valuable in influenza. A teaspoon of turmeric powder should be mixed in a cup of warm milk and taken three times a day. It will prevent complications arising from influenza, and also activate the liver which becomes sluggish during the attack.

Onion: Onion is also an effective remedy for influenza. Equal amounts of onion juice and honey should be mixed, and three or four teaspoons of this mixture should be taken daily in the treatment of this disease.

Ginger: Ginger is an excellent remedy for influenza. A teaspoon of fresh ginger juice, mixed with a cup of fenugreek decoction and honey to taste, is an excellent diaphoretic mixture which increases sweating and reduces fever in this disease. The fenugreek decoction may be prepared by boiling one tablespoon of fenugreek seeds in half a litre of water, till it is reduced by one-third.

Grapefruit: The juice of grapefruit has proved useful in this disease as it tones up the body and the digestive tract.

Basil Leaves: Another effective remedy for this disease is the green leaves of the basil plant. About one gram of these leaves should be boiled along with some ginger in half a litre of water till about half the water is left. This decoction should be taken as tea. It gives immediate relief.

Finger Millet: Fumigation of the burnt flour of finger millet is useful in influenza. It should be inhaled gently in the treatment of this disease. It will increase the blood circulation in the nasal mucosa, reduce local congestion, and open up the stuffed nose.

Dietary Considerations

In the acute stage of influenza, the patient should abstain from all solid foods and only drink fruit and vegetable juices diluted with water on a 50:50 basis for the first three to five days, depending on the severity of the condition. After the fever subsides, the patient may adopt an all-fruit diet for two or three days. This may be followed by a fruit and milk diet for a further two or three days. Thereafter, the patient may adopt a well-balanced diet of natural foods, with emphasis on fresh fruits and raw vegetables. He should avoid spices and condiments, alcohol, tobacco, strong tea and coffee, highly seasoned meats, over-boiled milk, pulses, potatoes, rice, cheese, and refined, processed, stale, and tinned foods.

Other Measures

A warm-water enema should be taken daily during the first three to five days of the treatment.

During the course of the fever, the natural way of reducing temperature is by means of cold body packs, which should be applied several times a day. The pack is made by wringing out a sheet or a large square piece of linen material in cold water, wrapping it right round the body and legs of the patient, and then covering it completely with a blanket. The pack can be kept for an hour or so, and the body should be sponged with tepid water after removing the pack. The patient should be kept in bed and should stay there till he is well again.

Insomnia

Inability to Sleep

The term insomnia literally denotes a complete lack of sleep. It is, however, used to indicate a relative inability to sleep that consists of difficulty in falling asleep, difficulty in remaining asleep, early final awakening, or combinations of these complaints. This disease has assumed alarming proportions in the present times, specially among the upper classes in the urban set-up.

Causes and Symptoms

The single symptom that most frequently marks the onset of insomnia is difficulty in falling asleep. There may be changes in the duration and quality of sleep, persistent changes in sleep patterns, lapses of memory, and lack of concentration during the day. Other symptoms are emotional instability, loss of coordination, and confusion.

The most common cause of sleeplessness is mental tension brought about by anxiety, worries, overwork, and overexcitement. Suppressed feelings of resentment, anger, and bitterness may also cause insomnia. Constipation, dyspepsia, overeating at night, excessive intake of tea or coffee, smoking, and going to bed hungry are among the other causes. Often, worrying about falling asleep is enough to keep one awake.

Remedies

Thiamine: Of the various food elements, thiamine or vitamin B_1 is of special significance in the treatment of insomnia. It is vital for strong, healthy nerves. A body starved of thiamine over a long period will be unable to relax and fall asleep naturally. Valuable sources of this vitamin are wholegrain cereals, pulses, and nuts.

Lettuce: Lettuce is beneficial in the treatment of insomnia as it contains a sleep-inducing substance, called 'lectucarium'. The juice of this plant has been likened in effect to the sedative action of opium without the accompanying excitement. Lettuce seeds taken in a decoction are also useful in insomnia. One tablespoon of seeds should be boiled in half a litre of water, till it is reduced by one-third.

Milk: Milk is very valuable in insomnia. A glass of milk, sweetened with honey, should be taken every night before going to bed in treating this condition. It acts as a tonic and a tranquilliser. Massaging the milk over the soles of the feet has also been found effective.

Curd: Curd is also useful in insomnia. The patient should take plenty of curd and massage it on the head. This will induce sleep.

Bottle Gourd: The mixture of bottle gourd juice and sesame oil in a 50:50 ratio acts as an effective medicine for insomnia. It should be massaged over the scalp every night. The cooked leaves of bottle gourd taken as a vegetable are also beneficial in the treatment of this disease.

Aniseed: A tea made from aniseed is valuable in sleeplessness. This tea is prepared by boiling about 375 ml of water in a vessel and adding a teaspoon of aniseed. The water should be covered with a lid and allowed to simmer for fifteen minutes. It should then be strained and drunk hot or warm. The tea may be sweetened with honey, and hot milk may also be added to it. This tea should be taken after meals or before going to bed.

Honey: Honey is beneficial in the treatment of insomnia. It has a hypnotic action and induces a sound sleep. It should be taken with water, before going to bed, in doses of two teaspoons in a large cup of water. Babies generally fall asleep after taking honey.

Rauwolfia: The herb rauwolfia is a valuable medicine for insomnia because of its indisputable efficacy as a sedative. The hypnotic action of the drug appears to have been known since ancient times. The very first dose of rauwolfia will enable a patient with a phlegmatic and gouty nature to go to sleep. The powder of the root in a quantity of 0.25 gm to 0.5 gm should be mixed with some scented substance like cardamom and given to the patient. The patient will have a sound sleep during the entire night. If the disease is chronic, the patient should take 0.25 gm twice a day, in the morning as well as at night before retiring.

Dietary Considerations

The patient should take a low-salt diet as salt is said to interfere with a restful sleep. A balanced diet with simple modifications in the eating pattern will go a long way in the treatment of insomnia. Such a diet should exclude white flour products, sugar and its products, tea, coffee, chocolate, cola drinks, alcohol, fatty foods, fried foods, and foods containing additives.

Other Measures

Regular active exercise during the day and mild exercise before retiring at night enhances the quantity and the quality of sleep. Yoga helps in a majority of cases. It provides physical and mental relaxation from one's disturbing problems. The traditional yoga *asanas* which are effective for insomnia patients are *shirshasana, sarvangasana, paschimottanasana, uttanasana, viparit karni,* and *shavasana.*

The patient should make an all-out effort to eliminate as many stress factors as possible. The steps in this direction should include regular practice of any relaxation method or meditation technique, cultivating the art of doing things slowly, particularly activities like eating, walking, and talking; limiting the working day to nine or ten hours and the working week to five and a half days; cultivating a creative hobby and spending some time daily on this; and avoiding meeting unrealistic targets.

Intestinal Worms

Hookworms, Roundworms,
Tapeworms, Threadworms

Worms and other intestinal parasites which infest human beings are found in all countries of the world. However, they are more common in tropical and subtropical areas and are widely prevalent during the rainy season. Children are more often infested with intestinal worms than adults.

Causes and Symptoms

The usual symptoms of intestinal worms are diarrhoea, foul breath, dark circles under the eyes, constant desire for food, restlessness at night with bad dreams, anaemia, and headaches. Round-worms may give rise to inflammation of the intestine and lungs, nausea, vomiting, loss of weight, fever, nervousness, and irritability. Threadworms may cause intense itching in the area around the rectum. They may also cause periodic bouts of diarrhoea alternating with constipation, loss of weight, cough, and fever. Hookworms may give rise to anaemia and nutritional disorders.

The eggs of these parasites are introduced into the human system through the medium of food or water. Roundworms are caused by eating contaminated food. Threadworms may enter the body from dirty fingers and food. Hookworms enter the human body through bare foot walking on infected earth. Tapeworms are transmitted to the body through undercooked flesh foods or foods contaminated by dogs.

The real cause of intestinal worms, however, is faulty living. The eggs of these worms, taken into the human body through food and water, can breed in the intestines only if they find there a suitable medium for their propagation. This medium is an intestinal tract clogged with morbid matter.

Remedies

Coconut: Among the numerous home remedies found beneficial in the treatment of intestinal worms, the use of coconut is most effective. It is an ancient remedy for expelling all kinds of intestinal worms. A tablespoon of freshly ground coconut should be taken at breakfast, followed by 30 to 60 ml of castor oil mixed with 250 to 375 ml of lukewarm milk after three hours. This process may be repeated till the cure is complete.

Garlic: Garlic has been used from ancient times by the Chinese, Greeks, Romans, Indians, and Babylonians for expelling intestinal worms. It is still used by modern medical practitioners for the same purpose. Both fresh garlic and its oil are effective. An ancient method of its administration was to place a couple of cloves of fresh garlic in each shoe. As the person walked, the cloves got crushed, and the worm-killing garlic oil was absorbed by the skin and carried by the blood into the intestines easily, as it possessed a powerful penetrative force. This ancient method is worth a trial by those who do not like the taste of garlic and cannot eat it. Those who can eat raw garlic, however, should chew three cloves of garlic every morning.

Carrot: Carrots are valuable in the elimination of threadworms among children as they are offensive to all parasites. A small cup of grated carrot taken every morning, with no other food added to the meal, can clear these worms quickly.

Papaya: The digestive enzyme papain in the milky juice of the unripe papaya is a powerful agent for destroying roundworms. A tablespoon of the fresh juice of an unripe papaya, and an equal quantity of honey should be mixed with three to four tablespoons of hot water and taken as a dose by an adult. This should be followed two hours later by a dose of 30 to 60 ml of castor oil mixed in 250–375 ml of lukewarm milk. This treatment should be repeated for two days if necessary. For children between seven to ten years of age, half the above doses should be given. For children under three years, a tablespoon is sufficient.

Papaya seeds are also useful for this purpose. They are rich in a substance called caricin which is a very effective medicine for expelling roundworms. The seeds should be powdered and taken in doses of one teaspoon with one cup of milk or water daily in the morning on an empty stomach. The alkaloid carpaine found in papaya leaves also has the power to destroy or expel intestinal worms. An infusion can be made by pouring 250 ml of boiling water over 15 gm of dry leaves. This can be taken with honey.

Pomegranate: The bark, both of the root and the stems of the pomegranate tree, is well known for its anthelmintic properties of destroying parasitic worms. The bark of the root is, however, preferred as it contains a greater quantity of the alkaloid punicine than the bark of the stem. This alkaloid is highly toxic to tapeworms. A cold decoction of the bark, preferably fresh bark, should be given in quantities of 90 to 180 ml three times, at intervals of one hour, to an adult. A purgative should be given after the last dose. The dose for children is 30 to 60 ml. The decoction is also used for expelling tapeworms.

Pumpkin: The seeds of ripe pumpkin are useful in intestinal worms, especially tapeworms. One tablespoon of the seeds should be peeled and crushed, and then infused in 250 ml of boiling water and drunk. This will kill the parasites and help in expelling the tapeworms. It will be necessary to fast for a day and empty the intestines by taking the juice of boiled dry prunes. The next day, three or four tumblers of the pumpkin seed infusion should be taken.

Wormwood: The herb wormwood is an ancient cure for expelling intestinal worms. It was extensively used by the Greeks and Romans for this purpose. The flowering tops have been and are, to this day, largely used in the Tibbi (Unani) system of medicine in India as a drug to kill intestinal worms. They are usually powdered and given in eight to sixteen gram doses daily for roundworms and tapeworms.

The oil distilled from this plant also possesses the property to kill worms. It should be mixed with olive oil, the latter being eight times the weight of the former. This mixture can be given in doses of 50 to 100 ml for this purpose. An infusion of the herb can also be prepared by mixing 2 ml of wormwood oil in 120 ml of water, and be given as an enema for killing worms in the rectum.

Belleric Myroblan: The herb belleric myroblan, mixed with the seeds of the herb butea *(palas)* on a 50:50 basis is an excellent anthelmintic. It should be given in doses of one teaspoon thrice a day. It helps remove all intestinal parasites. The seeds of butea can also be administered alone with beneficial results in expelling intestinal worms. One teaspoon of seeds may be given either in the form of powder or paste with one teaspoon of honey, thrice daily. They are specially beneficial in the treatment of roundworms and tapeworms.

Vasaka: The leaves, bark, root-bark, fruit, and the flowers of vasaka tree also help in removing intestinal parasites. A decoction of the root and bark can be prepared by boiling 30 gm of the root and bark in 500 ml of water, till it is reduced by one-third. This decoction may be given in doses of 30 ml twice or thrice daily for two or three days. The juice of the fresh leaves can also be used in doses of a teaspoon thrice a day for three days.

Calamus: Another valuable remedy for expelling intestinal worms is the herb calamus. The bitter element in this herb, acorin, is an anthelmintic.

Dietary Considerations

The treatment for intestinal worms should begin with diet. The patient should be kept on an exclusive fresh-fruit diet for four or five days. Thereafter, he may adopt a well-balanced light diet consisting mainly of fruits, vegetables, milk, and wholemeal bread. The diet should exclude fatty foods such as butter, cream, and oil, and all flesh foods.

In some cases, the all-fruit diet may have to be repeated at intervals and in obstinate cases, the patient should resort to a short fast of raw fruit and vegetable juices.

Other Measures

During the all-fruit or fasting period, the bowel should be cleansed daily with a warm-water enema.

Jaundice

Inflammation of the Liver

Jaundice is the most common of all liver disorders. It is a condition in which yellow discoloration of the skin and mucous membranes occur due to an increase in the bile pigments, namely, bilirubin, in the blood.

Causes and Symptoms

The symptoms of jaundice are extreme weakness, headache, fever, loss of appetite, severe constipation, nausea, and yellow discoloration of the eyes, tongue, skin, and urine. The patient may also feel a dull pain in the liver region. Obstructive jaundice may be associated with intense itching.

Jaundice may be caused by an obstruction of the bile ducts which normally discharge bile salts and pigment into the intestine. The bile gets mixed with blood and this gives a yellow pigmentation to the skin. The obstruction of the bile ducts could be due to gallstones or inflammation of the liver, which is known as hepatitis, and is caused by a virus. Other causes of jaundice are haemolytic anaemia and certain diseases affecting the liver such as typhoid, malaria, yellow fever, and tuberculosis.

Remedies

Bitter Luffa: The juice of bitter luffa is regarded as an effective remedy for jaundice. It is obtained by pounding and squeezing the bitter luffa through cloth. The juice should be placed on the palm of the hand and drawn up through the nostrils. This will cause a profuse outflow of a yellow-coloured fluid through the nostrils. The toxic matter having been evacuated in a considerable quantity, the patient will feel relieved. This is, however, a strong medicine and may cause side-effects like giddiness, migraine, and, at times, high fever for a short duration in patients with a delicate nature. Its use should, therefore, be avoided by such patients.

If the juice of green bitter luffa is not available, it can be substituted by two to three drops of the fluid obtained by soaking its dry crusts overnight in water. This will produce an identical effect. Seeds of bitter luffa which are easily available can also be used for the same purpose after rubbing in water.

Radish Leaves: The green leaves of radish are another valuable remedy for jaundice. The leaves should be pounded and their juice extracted through cloth. Half a litre of this juice should be taken daily by an adult patient. It induces a healthy appetite and proper evacuation of bowels, and this results in gradual decrease of the trouble. In most cases, complete cure can be ensured within eight or ten days.

Tomato: Tomatoes are valuable in jaundice. A glass of fresh tomato juice, mixed with a pinch of salt and pepper, taken early in the morning, is considered an effective remedy for this disease.

Snake Gourd Leaves: The leaves of snake gourd have also been found useful in jaundice. An infusion of the leaves should be prepared by mixing 15 gm of dry leaves in 250 ml of boiling water. Next, a decoction of coriander seeds can be prepared by boiling one tablespoon of coriander seeds in 500 ml of water till it is reduced by one-third. The infusion should be given in doses of 30 to 60 ml, mixed with the decoction of coriander seeds, thrice daily.

Pigeon Pea Leaves: The green leaves of pigeon pea, a leguminous plant – the beans of which are used for dals – are considered useful in jaundice. The juice extracted from these leaves should be taken in doses of 60 ml daily. Marked improvement will follow its use.

Almonds, Dried Dates and Cardamoms: A mixture of almonds, dried dates, and cardamoms is regarded as an effective remedy for jaundice. Eight kernels of almonds, two dried dates, and five small cardamoms should be soaked overnight in water. The outer coating of the almond kernels and the inner seeds of dried dates should be removed the next morning and the whole material should be rubbed into a fine paste. Then, fifty grams of sugar and an equal amount of butter should be mixed in it and the patient should lick this mixture.

Sugarcane Juice: One glass of sugarcane juice, mixed with the juice of half a lime, and taken twice daily, can hasten recovery from jaundice. It is, however, very essential that the juice must be clean and preferably prepared at home. Resistance is low in jaundice and any infected beverage could make matters worse.

Lemon: Lemon is also beneficial in the treatment of jaundice. The patient should be given 20 ml of lemon juice mixed with water several times a day. This will protect the damaged liver cells.

Barley Water: Barley water drunk several times during the day is another good remedy for this disease. One cup of barley should be boiled in three litres of water and simmered for three hours.

Jaundice Berry: The herb jaundice berry, botanically known as *Berberis vultaris* is very useful in jaundice. The pulverized bark should be given several times a day in doses of one-fourth of a teaspoon in the treatment of this disease, or the fluid extract should be given in 2–4 ml doses.

134

Dietary Considerations

A mild form of viral jaundice can be cured rapidly by diet therapy and physical rest. Recovery is, however, slow in jaundice caused by obstruction in the bile ducts, depending upon the cause and removal of the cause. The patient should be put on a juice fast for a week, and he should rest until the acute symptoms of the disease subside. After the juice fast, he may adopt an all-fruit diet for a further three to five days, taking three meals a day of fresh juicy fruits at five-hourly intervals. Thereafter, a simple light carbohydrate diet with exclusion of fats, best obtained from vegetables and fruits, may be resumed.

Digestive disturbances must be avoided. No food with a tendency to ferment or putrefy in the lower intestines like pulses and legumes should be included in the diet.

Other Measures

The patient should undertake only moderate exercise, fresh air baths, and adequate rest.

Kidney Stones

Pyelolithiasis

The formation of stones in the kidneys or urinary tract is not an uncommon disorder. The stones are formed from the chemicals usually found in the urine such as uric acid, phosphorus, calcium, and oxalic acid. They may vary in consistency from grit, sand, and gravel-like obstructions to the size of a bird's egg. Stones may form and grow because the concentration of a particular substance in the urine exceeds its solubility.

Most kidney stones are composed either of calcium oxalate or phosphate, the latter being most common in the presence of infection. About ninety per cent of all stones contain calcium as the chief constituent. More than half of these are mixtures of calcium, ammonium and magnesium, phosphates and carbonates, while the remainder contain oxalate.

Causes and Symptoms

Kidney stones usually cause severe pain in their attempt to pass down the ureter on their way to the bladder. The pain is first felt in the side and, thereafter, in the groin and thighs. Other symptoms of kidney stones are a frequent desire to urinate, painful urination, scanty urination, nausea, vomiting, sweating, and chills. The patient may also pass blood with the urine.

The formation of stones in the kidneys is the result of defects in the general metabolism. They usually occur when the urine becomes highly concentrated due to heavy perspiration or insufficient intake of fluids. They are aggravated by a sedentary life-style. The other causes are a wrong diet, excess intake of acid-forming foods, white flour and sugar products, meat, tea, coffee, condiments and spices, rich foods, and overeating. Lack of vitamin A and an excessive intake of vitamin D may also lead to formation of stones.

Remedies

Kidney Beans: Kidney beans, also known as dried French beans or *Rajmah*, are regarded as a very effective home remedy for kidney problems, including kidney stones. It was one Dr Ramm of Germany, who first discovered the value of kidney beans as a medicine for kidney and bladder troubles. He used it for over twenty-five years with beneficial results. The method prescribed by him to prepare the medicine is to remove the beans from inside the pods, then slice the pods and put about sixty grams in four litres of hot water, boiling them slowly for four hours. This liquid should be strained through fine muslin and then allowed to cool for about eight hours. Thereafter the fluid should be poured through another piece of muslin without stirring.

According to Dr Ramm, a glass of this decoction should be given to the patient every two hours throughout the day for one day and, thereafter, it may be taken several times a week. Dr Ramm also maintained that this decoction would not work if it was more than twenty-four hours old. The pods could be kept for longer periods but once they were boiled, the therapeutic factor would disappear after one day.[1]

Basil: Basil has a strengthening effect on the kidneys. In case of kidney stones, one teaspoon each of basil juice and honey

---

1. Quoted in Mark Bricklin's *Natural Home Remedies,* Rodale Press, India, 1986.

should be taken daily for six months. It has been found that stones can be expelled from the urinary tract by this treatment.

Celery: Celery is a valuable food for those who are prone to getting stones in the kidneys or gall-bladder. Its regular intake prevents future stone formation.

Apple: Apples are useful in kidney stones. In countries where the natural unsweetened cider is a common beverage, cases of stones or calculus are practically absent. The ripe fresh fruit is, however, more valuable.

Grapes: Grapes have an exceptional diuretic value on account of their high contents of water and potassium salt. The value of this fruit in kidney troubles is enhanced by its low albumin and sodium chloride content. It is an excellent cure for kidney stones.

Pomegranate: The seeds of both sour and sweet pomegranates are a useful medicine for kidney stones. A tablespoon of the seeds, ground into a fine paste, can be given along with a cup of horse gram *(kulthi)* soup to dissolve gravel in kidneys. Two tablespoons of horse gram should be used for preparing the cup of soup.

Watermelon: Watermelon contains the highest concentration of water amongst all fruits. It is also rich in potassium salts. It is one of the safest and best diuretics which can be used with beneficial results in kidney stones.

Vitamin B_6: Research has shown the remarkable therapeutic success of vitamin B_6 or pyridoxine in the treatment of kidney stones. A daily therapeutic dose of 100 to 150 mg of vitamin B_6, preferably combined with other B complex vitamins, should be continued for several months for getting a permanent cure.

Dietary Considerations

A patient with kidney stones should avoid foods which irritate the kidneys, to control acidity or alkalinity of the urine. He should also ensure adequate intake of fluids to prevent the urine from becoming concentrated. The foods considered irritants to the kidneys are alcoholic beverages; condiments and pickles; certain vegetables like cucumber, radish, tomato, spinach, rhubarb; those with a strong aroma such as asparagus, onion, beans, cabbage, and cauliflower; meat and gravies; and carbonated waters.

For controlling the formation of calcium phosphate stones, the intake of calcium and phosphates should be restricted. Foods which should be avoided are wholewheat flour, Bengal gram, peas, soyabean, beet, spinach, cauliflower, turnips, carrots, almonds, and coconuts.

When stones are composed of calcium, magnesium phosphates, and carbonates, the diet should be so regulated as to maintain an acidic urine. On the other hand, the urine should be kept alkaline if oxalate and uric acid stones are being formed. In the latter case, fruits and vegetables should be liberally used, and acid-forming foods should be kept to the minimum necessary for satisfactory nutrition. In case of uric stones, foods with a high purine content such as sweet breads, liver, and kidney should be avoided.

The patient should take a low-protein diet, restricting protein to one gram per kilogram of food. A liberal intake of fluid upto three litres or more daily is essential to prevent the precipitation of salts into the form of stones.

Other Measures

The patient should be given a large warm enema, followed by a hot bath with a temperature of 37.8^0C, gradually increased to 44.5^0C. During the bath, the head should be wrapped in a cold towel. Hot fomentation applied across the back in the region of the kidneys will relieve the pain. Certain *yogasanas* such as *pavanmuktasana, uttanpadasana, bhujangasana, dhanurasana,* and *halasana* are also beneficial as they activate the kidneys.

Leucoderma

White Patches on the Skin

Leucoderma, also known as vitiligo, is a distressing skin condition. The word literally means white skin. There is a gradual loss of the pigment melanin from the skin layers which results in white patches. These patches look ugly, especially in persons with a dark complexion. The condition does not cause any organic harm. This disease is caused neither by any germs, nor is it due to bad blood. It is considered to be neither infectious nor contagious.

Causes and Symptoms

The problem usually starts with a small white spot which later develops into patches. These patches are pale in the beginning, but become whiter and whiter as time passes by due to loss of pigment. As the spots enlarge, they merge into each other and, in course of time, form a very broad patch. In some cases, most of the skin of the body may be covered with white patches.

The main causes of leucoderma are said to be excessive mental worry, chronic or acute gastric disorders, impaired hepatic function such as jaundice, worms or other parasites in the alimentary canal, typhoid, a defective perspiratory mechanism, and burn injuries. Heredity is also a well-recognised causative factor.

Remedies

Psoralea: The best-known home remedy for leucoderma is the use of seeds of psoralea *(babchi)*. These seeds should be steeped in the juice of ginger for three days. The fluid should be renewed every day. The seeds should then be rubbed with the hands to remove the husks, dried in the shade and powdered. One gram of this powder should be taken every day with one cup of fresh milk for forty days continuously. The ground seeds should also be applied to the white spots.

Babchi seeds, combined with tamarind *(imli)* seeds, are also useful. An equal quantity of both the seeds should be steeped in water for three to four days. They should then be shelled and dried in the shade. They should be ground into paste and applied to the white patches for a week. If the application of this paste causes itching, or the white spots become red and a fluid begins to ooze out, this treatment should be discontinued.

Red Clay: Another useful remedy for leucoderma is red clay found by the river side or on hill slopes. The clay should be mixed in ginger juice in a ratio of 1:1, and applied over the white spots once a day. The copper contained in the clay seems to bring back skin pigmentation. Ginger juice also serves as a mild stimulant, facilitating increased blood flow to the spots. Drinking water kept overnight in a copper vessel will also help.

Radish: A paste made from the seeds of the radish is valuable in treating leucoderma. About thirty-five grams of these seeds should be powdered in two teaspoons of vinegar and applied on the white patches.

Goose Foot: The use of goose foot is beneficial in the treatment of this disease. This vegetable should be taken twice daily, in the morning as well as in the evening, for two months continuously. Simultaneously, the juice of the leaves should be applied over the patches of leucoderma.

Turmeric: Turmeric mixed with mustard oil has also proved useful in leucoderma. About 500 gm of turmeric should be pounded and soaked in 8 litres of water at night. It should be boiled in the morning till only one litre of water is left, and then be strained and mixed with 500 ml of mustard oil. This mixture should be heated till only the oil is left. It should then be strained and preserved in a bottle. The mixture should be applied on the white patches every morning and evening for a few months.

Dietary Considerations

Constitutional measures should be adopted to cleanse the system of accumulated toxins. To begin with, the patient should undertake a fast of juices for about a week. After the juice fast, the patient may adopt a restricted diet consisting of fresh fruits, raw or steamed vegetables, and wholemeal bread or *chapatis*. Curd and milk may be added to this diet after a few days. The patient may, thereafter, gradually embark upon a well-balanced diet of seeds, nuts, grains, vegetables, and fruits. This diet may be supplemented with cold-pressed vegetable oils, honey, and yeast. Juice fasting may be repeated at intervals of two months or so. The patient should avoid tea, coffee, alcoholic beverages, all condiments and highly-flavoured dishes, sugar, white flour products, denatured cereals like polished rice and pearled barley, and tinned or bottled foods.

Other Measures

During the initial one-week juice fast, the bowels should be cleansed daily with a lukewarm-water enema.

Leucorrhoea

White Vaginal Discharge

Leucorrhoea, commonly known as whites, refers to a whitish discharge from the female genitals. It is an abnormal disease condition of the reproductive organs of women. The condition may continue for weeks or months at a time. If not treated properly in the initial stages, it may become chronic.

Causes and Symptoms

In addition to the whitish discharge from the vagina, the patient feels weak and tired. She also suffers from pain in the lumbar region and the calves, and experiences a dragging sensation in the abdomen. Other symptoms are constipation, frequent headaches, and intense itching. In the chronic form, the patient feels irritable and develops black patches under the eyes.

Leucorrhoea denotes a generally devitalised and toxic condition of the system, caused by wrong feeding habits. Whenever the body is loaded with toxins and the eliminative organs such as the skin, bowels, lungs, and kidneys are unable to eliminate them, the body in women establishes profuse discharge or elimination through the mucous membrane of the uterus and vagina in the form of leucorrhoea. In young women, leucorrhoea may occur during inter-menstrual periods due to the thickening of the mucous membrane in the reproductive organs. During the child-bearing years from adolescence to the mid-forties, infection may sometimes follow the birth of a child due to damage of the cervix during delivery of the baby. The other common causes of leucorrhoea are displacement of the womb and unhygienic conditions which attract the bacteria to the genital organs.

Remedies

Amaranth Root: Amaranth is considered an excellent home remedy for leucorrhoea. The rind of the root of this plant should be rubbed in 25 ml of water. It should then be strained and given to the patient daily in the morning as well as in the evening. The root of this plant is, however, very susceptible to moths. Hence, care should be taken to see that it is not moth-eaten. In case the root is not available, its leaves and branches may be similarly processed and used.

Lady's Fingers: The use of lady's fingers is another effective home remedy for this disease. A decoction of this vegetable is prepared by boiling 100 gm of the fresh vegetable, cut transversely, in half a litre of water for twenty minutes. It should then be strained and sweetened. This decoction, given in doses of 60 to 90 ml frequently, is beneficial in all irritable conditions of genito-urinary organs, including leucorrhoea.

Fenugreek Seeds: Fenugreek seeds are valuable in leucorrhoea. They should be taken internally in the form of tea and also used as a douche. For a douche, the solution should be much stronger than tea. Two tablespoons of fenugreek seeds should be put into a litre of cold water and allowed to simmer for half an hour over a low flame. The decoction should then be strained and used as a douche.

Guava Leaves: The tender leaves of guava are beneficial in the treatment of this disease. An infusion of the leaves should be used as a douche. It acts as a powerful vaginal astringent.

Mango Seed: Mango seeds are valuable in leucorrhoea. A teaspoon of the paste of the decorticated kernel of mango can be applied inside the vagina with beneficial results.

Walnut Leaves: The leaves of the walnut tree contain astringent chemicals. A decoction of the fresh leaves can be beneficially used as a douche in the treatment of leucorrhoea.

Dietary Considerations

To begin with, the patient should fast for three or four days on fruit juices for the elimination of the morbid matter. After a short juice fast, she may adopt an all-fruit diet for about a week, taking three meals a day of fresh juicy fruits. The patient may, thereafter, gradually embark upon a well-balanced diet, with emphasis on wholegrain cereals, fresh fruits, and raw and steamed vegetables. She should avoid all forms of white flour, white sugar, fried and greasy foods, condiments, preserves, tea, and coffee.

Other Measures

Water treatment is extremely beneficial in curing leucorrhoea. A cold hip bath taken twice a day, for ten minutes at a time, will help relieve congestion in the pelvic region and facilitate quick elimination of morbid matter. A warm vaginal douche at 30^0 C to 40^0C is beneficial for general cleaning and elimination of the purulent discharge. The procedure is to fill the douche can with one and a half litres of warm water and hang it at a level of three feet above the body. The patient should lie with the hips slightly raised above the body level, and the special nozzle applied for this purpose should be oiled and inserted slowly into the vagina. The flow can be regulated by the small valve of the nozzle. In severe cases, the douche should be taken daily.

Loss of Hair

Although hair is not essential to life, it is of sufficient cosmetic concern to provoke anxiety in anyone when it starts thinning, falling, or disappearing. To a woman, the sight of a comb or brush covered with lost hair can cause intense mental strain.

Hair is formed in minute pockets in the skin called follicles. An upgrowth at the base of the follicle, called the papilla, actually produces hair when a special group of cells turn amino acids into keratin, a type of protein of which hair is made. The rate of production of these protein 'building blocks' determines hair growth. The average growth rate is about 1.2 cm per month, growing fastest on women between fifteen to thirty years of age.

Causes and Symptoms

The most important cause of loss of hair is inadequate nutrition. Even a partial lack of almost any nutrient may cause hair to fall. Persons lacking in vitamin B_6 lose their hair and those deficient in folic acid often become completely bald. But the hair grows normally after the liberal intake of these vitamins. Other important causes of loss of hair are stress such as worry, anxiety, and sudden shock; general debility caused by severe or long standing illnesses like typhoid, syphilis, chronic cold, influenza, and anaemia, an unclean condition of the scalp which weakens the hair roots by blocking the pores with the collected dirt; and heredity.

Remedies

Rubbing of Scalp: A vigorous rubbing of the scalp with fingers after washing the hair with cold water is one of the most effective among the several home remedies for the prevention and treatment of loss of hair. The scalp should be rubbed vigorously till it starts to tingle with the heat. It will activate the sebaceous glands and energise the circulation of blood in the affected area, making the hair grow healthy.

***Amla* Oil:** *Amla* oil, prepared by boiling the dry pieces of *amla* in coconut oil, is considered a valuable hair tonic for enriching hair growth. A mixture of an equal quantity of fresh *amla* juice and lime juice, used as a shampoo, also stimulates hair growth and prevents hair loss.

Lettuce: Lettuce is useful in preventing hair loss. A mixture of lettuce and spinach juice is believed to help the growth of hair if taken to the extent to half a litre a day.

Amaranth: Amaranth is another valuable remedy for loss of hair. Its fresh leaf juice should be applied to the hair. It will help the growth of the hair and keep it soft.

Alfalfa: The juice of alfalfa, in combination with equal quantities of carrot and lettuce juices, taken daily, also helps the growth of hair to a remarkable extent. The combination of these juices is rich in elements which are particularly useful for the growth of hair. While preparing alfalfa juice, the leaves of the plant may be used when they can be obtained fresh.

Margosa: The leaves of the margosa tree are also beneficial in the treatment of loss of hair. If the hair has been falling or has ceased to grow, it should be washed with the decoction of *neem* leaves. This will stop the hair from falling and stabilise its blackness. It will also make the hair longer and kill lice and other infesting insects.

Mustard Oil and Henna Leaves: Mustard oil, boiled with henna leaves, is useful for healthy growth of hair. About 250 ml of mustard oil should be boiled in a tin basin. About sixty grams of henna leaves should be gradually put in this oil till they are burnt in the oil. The oil should then be filtered through a cloth and stored well in a bottle. Regular massage of the head with this oil will produce abundant hair.

Coconut Milk: The application of coconut milk all over the scalp and massaging it into the hair roots is also beneficial in the treatment of loss of hair. It nourishes the hair and promotes hair growth. Coconut milk is prepared by grinding the coconut shavings and squeezing them well.

Lime-Pepper Seeds: Certain home remedies have also been found beneficial in the treatment of patchy baldness. The most valuable of these remedies is the seeds of lime and black pepper, ground together to get a fine paste. This paste applied on the patches, has a mildly irritant action. This increases blood circulation to the affected area and stimulates hair growth. The paste should be applied twice a day, for a few weeks.

Liquorice: The paste of liquorice, made by grinding the pieces in milk with a pinch of saffron, is another valuable remedy for patchy baldness. This paste should be applied over the bald patches at night before going to bed.

Onion: Onion has also been found beneficial in patchy baldness. The affected part should be rubbed with onions morning and evening till it is red. It should be rubbed with honey afterwards.

Pigeon Pea: A fine paste made from pigeon pea or red gram can also be applied regularly on bald patches for beneficial results.

Other Remedies: Daily application of refined coconut oil, mixed with lime water and lime juice, on the hair, prevents loss of hair and lengthens it. Application of the juice of green coriander leaves on the head is also considered beneficial.

Washing the hair with a paste of cooked black gram *(urad dal)* and fenugreek *(methi)* lengthens the hair. Regular use of castor oil as hair oil helps the luxuriant growth of the hair.

Dietary Considerations

The healthy condition of the hair depends, to a very large extent, on the intake of sufficient amounts of essential nutrients in the daily diet. Persons with a tendency to lose hair should take a well-balanced and correct diet, made up of foods which, in combination, should supply all the essential nutrients. It has been found that a diet which contains liberal quantities of seeds, nuts, grains, vegetables, and fruits would provide adequate amounts of all the essential nutrients. Each food group should roughly form the bulk of one of the three principal meals. These foods should, however, be supplemented with certain special foods such as milk, vegetable oils, honey, wheat germ, yeast, and liver.

Other Measures

Proper cleaning of the hair, and rubbing of the scalp with a towel after a hairwash, are necessary.

Low Blood Pressure

Hypotension

Low blood pressure or hypotension refers to the fall in blood pressure below normal. It is a condition in which the action of the heart, in forcing the blood through the arteries, is weak. This is a direct outcome of a weakened and devitalised system.

Causes and Symptoms

The patient with chronic low blood pressure may complain of lethargy, weakness, fatigue, and dizziness. The patient may faint, especially if arterial pressure is lowered further when he assumes an erect position. These symptoms are presumably due to a decrease in perfusion of blood to the brain, heart, skeletal muscle, and other organs.

The most important cause of low blood pressure is faulty nutrition. It makes the tissues forming the walls of the blood vessels over-relaxed, and flabby or streched. This results in less supply of oxygen and nutrients to the tissues. Malnutrition can result from a diet deficient in calories, proteins, vitamin C, or almost any one of the B vitamins.

Sometimes the blood pressure falls rapidly because of loss of blood. Low blood pressure may also develop gradually because of slow bleeding in the gastrointestinal tract, kidneys, or bladder. Emotional problems are a far more frequent cause of low blood pressure. To a lesser degree, prolonged disappointment and frustration may result in a subnormal blood pressure.

Remedies

Beetroot: The juice of raw beetroot is one of the most effective home remedies for low blood pressure. The patient should drink a cup of this juice twice daily for treating this condition. Considerable improvement will be noticeable within a week.

Indian Spikenard: The herb Indian spikenard is another effective home remedy for low blood pressure. It should be taken in doses of thirty to forty grains with a pinch of a little camphor and cinnamon *(dalchini)*. An infusion can also be prepared by steeping 15 to 20 gm of the herb in 250 ml of boiling water, and taking it thrice a day.

Nutrients: Protein, vitamin C, and all vitamins of the B group have been found beneficial in the prevention and treatment of low blood pressure. Of these, pantothenic acid is of particular importance. Liberal use of this vitamin alone often helps in raising the blood pressure. A diet which contains adequate quantities of complete proteins, B vitamins and, particularly, the nutrients that stimulate adrenal production, quickly normalizes low blood pressure.

Salt: The use of salt is valuable in low blood pressure. Until the blood pressure reaches normal levels through proper dietary and other remedies, it is essential that the patient should take salty foods and half a teaspoon of salt in water daily.

Epsom Salts Bath: Hot Epsom salts baths are one of the simplest remedies for low blood pressure. An Epsom salts bath is prepared by dissolving one to one and a half kg of commercial Epsom salts in an ordinary bath of hot water. The patient should remain immersed in the bath for ten to twenty minutes. This bath should be taken just before retiring to bed, and care should be exercised not to catch a chill afterwards.

Dietary Considerations

The treatment for low blood pressure should aim at rejuvenation of the whole system. To begin with, the patient should adopt an exclusive fresh fruit diet for about five days, taking three meals a day of fresh juicy fruits at five-hourly intervals. Thereafter, he may adopt a fruit and milk diet for two or three weeks. After the fruit and milk diet, the patient may gradually embark upon a well-balanced diet, consisting of seeds, nuts, and grains, with emphasis on fresh fruits and raw vegetables. Further periods of an all-fruit diet followed by a milk and fruit diet may be necessary every two or three months in some cases, depending on the progress being made.

Other Measures

A warm-water enema should be used daily to cleanse the bowels during the first few days of the treatment, and afterwards, if necessary. Those who are habitually constipated should take all possible steps for its eradication.

Daily dry friction and sponging should be undertaken by those suffering from low blood pressure. They should also undertake breathing and other light exercises like walking, swimming, and cycling. The patient should take sun and air baths and spend as much time as possible in the fresh air.

All living habits which tend to enervate the system, such as overwork, excesses of all kinds, needless worry, and negative thinking must be eliminated as far as possible.

Low Blood Sugar

Low blood sugar or hypoglycaemia is a disorder of blood sugar metabolism.

Causes and Symptoms

A craving for sweets and starch in excessive amounts between meals is the first sign of a low blood sugar level. When the blood sugar level falls much below normal, symptoms such as nervousness, irritability, fatigue, depression, disturbed vision, and headaches appear. Other symptoms are sweating, trembling, numbness, absent-mindedness, dizziness, palpitations of the heart, and some sexual disturbances. Most hypoglycaemia patients feel hungry and eat frequently to get over the feeling of weakness and emotional irritability. They feel tense if they have to go without food for several hours. Low blood sugar can compound into an emergency condition. In such an eventuality, medical help should be sought immediately. However, when the patient experiences any symptoms that indicate a fall in blood sugar, he should immediately take a heaped teaspoonful of sugar and then seek medical help.

Low blood sugar is usually caused by an excessive intake of refined carbohydrates and sugary foods. These substances cause the pancreas, the adrenal glands, and the liver to lose their ability to handle the sugar properly. Other causes of low blood sugar are a tumour; or a disturbed functioning of the liver, pituitary gland, or adrenal glands. Stress intensifies this condition.

Remedies

Vitamins: Certain vitamins have been found effective in the treatment of low blood sugar. These are vitamins C, E, and B complex. Foods rich in these vitamins are therefore valuable in low blood sugar. Vitamins C and B increase tolerance of sugar and carbohydrates, and help normalise sugar metabolism. Pantothenic acid and vitamin B_6 help to build up adrenals which are generally exhausted in persons with low blood sugar. Vitamin E improves glycogen storage in the muscles and tissues. The patient should take vitamin C in large doses from 2,000 to 5,000 mg, B_6 – 50 mg, and vitamin E – upto 1,600 IU daily.

Apple: Apples are considered valuable in low blood sugar. Two small apples with their peels should be taken after each meal for treating this condition.

Molasses: The use of molasses has been found very useful in low blood sugar. When blood sugar becomes abnormally low as a result of over exertion or under-nutrition, a glass of sherbet made of molasses will serve as a tonic and prevent the feeling of faintness. It serves the same purpose in the body as glucose.

Dietary Considerations

The ideal diet for low blood sugar should be based on three basic food groups, namely, grains, seeds and nuts, vegetables and fruits; supplemented by milk and milk products, and vegetable oils. Seeds, nuts, and grains should be the main constituents of the diet. Seeds and nuts should be taken in their raw form. Grains, in the form of cereals, should be cooked. Cooked grains are digested slowly and release sugar into the blood gradually, six to eight hours after meals. This will keep the blood sugar level normal and constant for a long period.

Persons suffering from a low blood sugar should take six to eight meals a day instead of two or three large ones. Eating raw nuts and seeds such as pumpkin or sunflower seeds, or drinking milk, buttermilk, or fruit juices between meals will be beneficial. All refined and processed foods, white sugar, white flour and all their by-products should be completely eliminated from the diet. Coffee, alcohol, and soft drinks should also be avoided. The consumption of salt should be reduced as an excessive intake of salt causes loss of blood potassium, which causes blood sugar to drop.

Other Measures

Proper rest is essential for those suffering from low blood sugar. A tranquil mind is of utmost importance in this condition. Nervous strain and anxiety should be relieved by simple methods of meditation and relaxation. *Yogasanas* like *vakrasana, bhujangasana, halasana, sarvangasana;* and pranayama like *kapalbhati* and *anuloma-viloma* will be beneficial. A prolonged bath at room temperature will also be helpful in relieving mental tension.

Malaria

Malaria is one of the most widespread diseases in the world, especially in tropical and subtropical regions.

Causes and Symptoms

There are three main types of malaria, depending upon the parasites which cause it. They are tertian fever, quartan fever and malignant tertian malaria. The most common symptom of all types of malaria is high fever, which may occur every day, on alternate days, or every fourth day. The fever is accompanied by chills, headache, shivering, and pain in the limbs. The temperature comes down after some time with profuse sweating. The main complications of malaria are anaemia, kidney failure, and dysentery.

Malaria is caused by a tiny parasite called *Plasmodium*. The parasite grows in the liver of a person for a few days and then enters the bloodstream where it invades the red blood cells. The disease spreads from a sick person to a healthy one by the bite of an infected female anopheles mosquito. She draws a small quantity of blood containing the parasites when she bites a person who has malaria. These parasites then pass through several stages of development within the mosquito's body, and finally find their way to its salivary glands. There they lie in wait for an opportunity to enter the bloodstream of the next person the mosquito bites. The malaria-carrying mosquito breeds in stagnant water.

According to naturopathy, however, the real causes of malaria are wrong feeding habits and a faulty style of living, which result in the system being clogged with accumulated systemic refuse and morbid matter. It is on this soil that the malaria germ breeds. The liberal intake of flesh foods, tinned and other denatured foods, and alcoholic beverages lowers the vitality of the system and paves the way for the development of malaria.

Remedies

Grapefruit: Grapefruit is one of the most effective home remedies for malaria. It should be taken daily. It contains a natural quinine-like substance which can be extracted from the fruit by boiling a quarter of a grapefruit and straining its pulp.

Fever Nut: The seeds of the fever nut plant are another effective remedy for malaria. They can be obtained from a herbal store and preserved in a phial for use when required. About six grams of these seeds should be given with a cup of water two hours before the expected onset of the paroxysm of fever, and a second dose should be given one hour after the attack. The paroxysm can thus be avoided but even if it occurs, the same procedure should be resorted to on that day and it will cut short the fever.

Datura: The leaves of the datura plant are useful in the tertian type of malarial fever. About two and a half freshly-sprouted leaves of this plant should be made into a pill by rubbing them with jaggery and administered two hours before the onset of the paroxysm.

Cinnamon: Cinnamon is regarded as a valuable remedy in malaria. One teaspoon should be coarsely powdered and boiled in a glass of water with a pinch of pepper powder and honey. This can be used beneficially as a medicine in malaria.

Chirayata: The herb *chirayata*, botanically known as *Swertia chirata*, is also beneficial in the treatment of intermittent malarial fevers. It helps in lowering the temperature. An infusion of the herb, prepared by steeping 15 gm of *chirayata* in 250 ml of hot water with aromatics like cloves and cinnamon, should be given in doses of 15 to 30 ml.

Lime and Lemon: Lime and lemon are valuable in the quartan type of malarial fever. About three grams of lime should be dissolved in about 60 ml of water and the juice of one lemon added to it. This water should be taken before the onset of the fever.

Alum: Alum is also useful in malaria. It should be roasted over a hot plate and powdered. Half a teaspoon should be taken about four hours before the expected attack and half a teaspoon every two hours after it. This will give relief.

Holy Basil: The leaves of holy basil are considered beneficial in the prevention of malaria. An infusion of a few leaves can be taken daily for this purpose. The juice of about eleven grams of leaves of holy basil mixed with three grams of powder of black pepper can be taken beneficially in the cold stage of the malarial fever. This will check the severity of the disease.

Dietary Considerations

Diet is of utmost importance in the treatment of malaria. To begin with, the patient should fast on orange juice and water for a few days, depending on the severity of the fever.

After the fever has subsided, the patient should be placed on an exclusive fresh-fruit diet for the first few days. Milk may then be added to the diet. Thereafter, the patient may gradually embark upon a well-balanced diet of natural foods, with emphasis on fresh fruits, and raw vegetables.

Other Measures

A warm-water enema should be administered daily during the juice and water fast to cleanse the bowels.

The best way to reduce temperature naturally during the course of the fever is by means of a cold pack, which can be applied to the whole body. This pack is made by wringing out a sheet or any other large square piece of linen material in cold water, wrapping it right round the body and legs of the patient (twice round would be best), and then covering it completely with a small blanket or similar warm material. This pack should be applied every three hours during the day while the temperature is high and kept on for an hour or so. Hot-water bottles may be kept on the feet and against the sides of the body.

Malaria can be prevented by protection against mosquito bites, cleanliness of surrounding areas, and ensuring that there is no pool of stagnant water lying around.

Measles

Skin Rash (Morbilli) and Fever

Measles, a highly infectious disease, is very common in childhood. It is so common at this stage of life that nearly all children in most parts of the world suffer from it.

Causes and Symptoms

The first symptoms that appear for seven to fourteen days after exposure to the virus are feverishness, cold, watering of the eyes, and a dry cough. A rash appears on the skin four days after the onset of these symptoms. This rash, which consists of small rounded

152

spots with reddened skin in between, initially appears on the sides of the face and the neck, and then gradually spreads all over the body, appearing last on the extremities. Initially pink in colour, the spots grow darker as time passes.

Measles is usually accompanied by fever and diarrhoea. In severe cases, high fever and delirium may occur. Complications which can arise from this disease include pneumonia, bronchitis, and abscesses in the ears. One serious but rare complication is inflammation of the brain.

Measles is one of the most contagious diseases caused by a virus. This disease is easily transmitted in the early stages through the invisible droplets of moisture which are discharged from a patient's nose or mouth when he coughs or sneezes. The real causes of this disease, like other diseases of childhood, are however, wrong feeding habits and unhygienic living conditions.

Remedies

Orange: Oranges are very valuable in measles, as the digestive power of the body is seriously hampered. The patient suffers from intense toxaemia, and the lack of saliva coats his tongue and often destroys his thirst for water as well as his desire for food. The agreeable flavour of orange juice helps greatly in overcoming these drawbacks. Orange juice is the ideal liquid food for this disease.

Lemon Juice: The juice of lemon also makes an effective thirst-quenching drink in measles. About 15 to 25 ml of lemon juice, diluted with water, should be taken for this purpose.

Turmeric: Turmeric is beneficial in the treatment of measles. Raw roots of turmeric should be dried in the sun and ground to a fine powder. Half a teaspoon of this powder, mixed with a few drops of honey and the juice of a few bitter gourd leaves, should be given to patients suffering from measles.

Liquorice: Powdered liquorice has been found valuable in relieving the cough, which is typical in measles. The child patient should be given half a teaspoon of powdered liquorice mixed with the same quantity of honey.

Barley: The use of barley water has proved beneficial for the troublesome cough in measles. This water should be taken frequently, sweetened with the newly-drawn oil of sweet almonds.

Egg Plant Seeds: The seeds of the egg plant are a stimulant. Intake of half to one gram of these seeds daily for three days will help develop immunity against measles for one year.

Dietary Considerations

At the beginning of the treatment, the patient should be given juices of fresh fruits like oranges and lemons frequently. This is sufficient as the child suffers from a lack of appetite during this period.

As the condition improves, the child can be placed on an all-fruit diet for a few days. Thereafter he may be allowed to gradually embark upon a well-balanced diet.

Other Measures

The child should be kept in a well-ventilated room. As light has a detrimental effect upon the eyes during measles because of the weakened condition of the external eye tissues, the child should have his eyes shaded or the room should have subdued light.

The treatment should aim at bringing down the temperature and eliminating the toxins from the system. This can be achieved by administration of a warm-water enema every morning, application of mud packs on the abdomen twice a day — in the morning and evening, and repeated application of chest packs. Lukewarm water baths can be given every day to ease itching. Addition of extracts of *neem* leaves to this water will prove beneficial.

Children having measles should not be allowed to mix with others so as to avoid passing on the infection to them. In fact, they should take complete rest. Hygienic conditions, along with the above-mentioned treatment, will lead to a speedy recovery. Medication should be strictly avoided.

Menopausal Disorders

Disorders Related to Cessation of Menses

Menopause or cessation of menses in women is a normal event which occurs in the mid or late forties. It signifies the end of the female reproductive period of life, which commences at adolescence in the early teens.

Causes and Symptoms

At the time of menopause, the entire chain of endocrine glands is affected, particularly, the gonads, thyroid, and pituitary glands.

In some women, the menopausal change takes place without any unpleasant symptoms, the only change really being the cessation of menstrual flow. There are, however, many women who develop disturbing symptoms such as hot flushes, night sweats, tension, insomnia, diminished interest in sex, irritability, and depression. Other symptoms are fatigue, palpitations, dizziness, headaches, and numbness.

Disturbing symptoms associated with menopause arise from the fact that the ovaries are no longer producing their normal amount of estrogen, the dominant female hormone. Anything which interferes with the normal functioning of the ovaries may also bring about these symptoms. Lack of a normal hormonal balance may also result in a severe backache which is caused by thinning of the bones. This condition is called osteoporosis and arises from the low level of estrogen in the bloodstream.

Remedies

Nutrients: During menopause, lack of ovarian hormones can result in severe calcium deficiency. For this reason, a larger than usual intake of calcium may help greatly. Vitamin D is also essential for assimilation of calcium. Any woman experiencing disturbing symptoms at this time should supplement her daily diet with 1,000 units of natural vitamin D, 500 mg of magnesium, and obtain 2 gm of calcium daily which can be supplied by one litre of milk.

Beet Juices: Beet juice has been found very useful in menopausal disorders. It should be taken in small quantities of 60 to 90 ml at a time, thrice a day. It has proved much more permanently helpful than the degenerative effects of drugs or synthetic hormones.

Carrot Seeds: Carrot seeds have also been found valuable in menopausal tension. A teaspoon of the seeds should be boiled in a glass of cow's milk for about ten minutes and taken daily as a medicine in the treatment of this condition.

Liquorice: The use of liquorice is one of the most effective remedies for menopausal disorders. Liquorice contains the natural female hormone, estrogen, and can, to some degree, compensate for the diminished hormone. One teaspoon of the powder should be taken daily.

Indian Spikenard: The herb Indian spikenard is another valuable remedy for certain disturbances due to menopause. It should be given in small doses of 2 gm daily. It will soothen the nervous system and induce tranquillity of the mind.

Dietary Considerations

Diet is of utmost importance in menopausal disorders. It should comprise of seeds, nuts, grains, vegetables, and fruits, with emphasis on vitamin E—rich foods, raw and sprouted seeds and nuts, unpasturised high-quality milk, and homemade cottage cheese. An abundance of raw, organically grown fruits and vegetables should be included in the diet. Plenty of freshly-made juices of fruits and vegetables in season should be included. All processed, refined, and denatured foods should be completely eliminated.

Other Measures

Plenty of outdoor exercise such as walking, jogging, swimming, horse-riding, or cycling are imperative. Other helpful measures in this direction are avoidance of mental and emotional stresses and worries, especially worry about getting old; sufficient sleep and relaxation; and following all the general rules of maintaining a high level of health.

Menstrual Problems

Problems Related to Menses

The two major female sex hormones in the body are estrogen and progesterone. They are produced in a pair of organs in the abdomen, known as the ovaries. The ovaries start producing large quantities of estrogen when a girl reaches about 12 years of age. This enables her to grow rapidly and develop into a normal young woman. The commencement of menstruation at this time heralds the reproductive phase of her life, when she can have children.

The main problems relating to menstrual flow are pre-menstrual tension, painful menstruation, stoppage of menstruation, and excessive menstruation. These disorders are not uncommon.

Causes and Symptoms

Premenstrual Tension and Menstrual Cramps: A few days before menstruation, some women become nervous and irritable. They suffer from depression, headaches, fullness in the breasts, insomnia, and swelling in the lower extremities. This may be due to a hormonal imbalance. These problems cease within twenty-four hours of the start of the menstrual flow.

Dysmenorrhoea: Painful menstruation, as it is called in medical parlance, is a common condition. The pain may be felt either two or three days before or immediately before or during the flow. This may also be due to a hormonal imbalance.

Amenorrhoea or Stoppage of Menstrual Flow: This is natural during pregnancy and at the menopause, but abnormal at any other time. It denotes a debilitated and devitalised condition of the body. The main causes contributing towards this condition are anaemia, worry, grief, fright, or other serious emotional disturbances; malformation of the womb; tuberculosis; displacement of the womb; and debility, especially after a serious illness.

Menorrhagia or Excessive Menstrual Flow: This is common in some women. A variety of causes may be responsible for this trouble, including fibroids.

Remedies

Parsley: Parsley is one of the most effective among the several home remedies in the treatment of menstrual disorders. It increases menstruation and assists in the regularization of the monthly periods. This action is due to the presence of apiol, which is a constituent of the female sex hormone oestrogen. Cramps, which are a result of menstrual irregularities, are relieved and frequently corrected entirely by the regular use of parsley juice, particularly in conjunction with beet juice; or with beet, carrot, and cucumber juices. The recommended quantity is 75 ml of each of the four juices.

Ginger: The use of ginger is another effective home remedy for menstrual disorders, especially in cases of painful menstruation and stoppage of menstrual flow. A piece of fresh ginger should be pounded and boiled in a cup of water for a few minutes. The infusion, sweetened with sugar, should be used thrice daily after meals as a medicine for treating this condition.

Sesame Seeds: Sesame seeds are valuable in menstrual problems. Half a teaspoon of powder of these seeds, taken with hot water twice daily, acts excellently in reducing spasmodic pain during menstruation in young, unmarried anaemic girls. Its regular use, two days prior to the expected periods, cures scanty menstruation. A warm hip bath containing a handful of crushed sesame seeds should be simultaneously taken along with this recipe.

Papaya: The unripe papaya helps the contractions of the muscle fibres of the uterus and is thus beneficial in securing a proper menstrual flow. Papaya is especially helpful when menstruation ceases due to stress or fright in young unmarried girls.

Bengal Gram: A bath prepared by putting an entire Bengal gram plant in hot water is beneficial in painful menstruation. The plant also may be used for a sitting steam bath.

Marigold: The herb Marigold, named after the Virgin Mary, is useful in allaying any pain during menstruation and facilitating menstrual flow. An infusion of the herb should be given in doses of one tablespoon twice daily for the treatment of these disorders.

Banana Flower: The use of banana flower is one of the most effective home remedies in the treatment of menorrhagia or excessive menstruation. One banana flower should be cooked and eaten with one cup of curd. This will increase the quantity of progesterone and reduce the bleeding.

Coriander Seeds: Coriander seeds are also beneficial in the treatment of excessive menstruation. Six grams of these seeds should be boiled in half a litre of water. This decoction should be taken off the fire when only half the water remains. Sugar candy should be added to it and the patient should drink it when it is still warm.

Mango Bark: The juice of the fresh mango bark is another valuable remedy for heavy bleeding during menstruation. The juice is given with the addition of white of an egg or some mucilage — a kind of vegetable glue obtained from a plant, and a small quantity of the kernel of a poppy. As an alternative, a mixture of 10 ml of a fluid extract of the bark, and 120 ml of water may be given in doses of one teaspoon every hour or two.

Ashoka: The bark of the *Ashoka* tree is an effective remedy for excessive blood loss during the monthly period which occurs due to uterine fibroids and other causes. It should be given in the form of decoction in treating this condition.

About 90 gm of the bark should be boiled in 30 ml of milk and 360 ml of water till the total quantity is reduced to about 90 gm. This quantity should be given in one day, in two or three doses. The treatment should commence from the fourth day of the monthly period and should be continued till the bleeding is checked. A fresh decoction should be made for use each day.

Indian Barbery: The herb Indian barbery is also useful in case of excessive bleeding. It should be given in doses of thirteen to twenty-five grams daily.

Rough Chaff: The herb rough chaff is also valuable in excessive menstruation. An infusion of the herb should be prepared by steeping 15 gm of rough chaff in 250 ml of water and used for treating this condition.

Hermal: The herb hermal is useful in regulating the menstrual periods. It is especially beneficial in painful and difficult menstruation. Two tablespoons of the seeds should be boiled in half a litre of water, till it is reduced by one - third. This decoction should be given in 15 to 30 ml doses.

Hemp: Hemp can be successfully used when menses do not start at the scheduled time. Five large heads of hemps should be boiled in half a litre of water till the water is reduced to half. It should then be strained and drunk before going to bed for two or three nights. This remedy seldom fails.

Dietary Considerations

The various disorders relating to menstrual flow, being systemic in origin, can be tackled only by treating the system as a a whole, so as to remove the toxicity from the body and build up the general health level of the sufferer. To undertake such a scheme of all-round, health-building treatment, the sufferer should begin with an all-fruit diet for about five days, taking three meals a day of fresh, juicy fruits. However, if there is excessive weight loss during the all-fruit diet, those already underweight may add a glass of milk to each fruit meal. After the all-fruit diet, the sufferer should adopt a well-balanced diet, with emphasis on fresh fruits, raw vegetables, and wholegrain cereals. The foods which should be avoided are white flour products, sugar, confectionery, rich cakes, pastries, sweets, refined cereals, greasy foods, tinned or preserved foods, strong tea, coffee, pickles, and condiments.

Further short periods of all-fruit fasts for two or three consecutive days, can be undertaken at monthly intervals, according to the need of the case.

Other Measures

During the first five days of an all-fruit diet, the bowels should be cleansed daily with a warm-water enema. Dry friction and a cold hip bath should form a regular feature of the treatment every morning. All cold baths should, however, be suspended during the menstrual period.

Smoking, if habitual, should be given up completely as it aggravates menstrual disorders.

Migraine

Severe Headache with Nausea

Migraine can be defined as a paroxysmal ailment, accompanied by a severe headache, generally on one side of the head, and associated with disorders of the digestion, the liver, and the vision. It usually occurs when a person is under great mental tension or has suddenly got over that state.

Persons who suffer from this disease have a particular type of personality. They are intelligent, sensitive, rigid, and methodical, and tend to be perfectionists. A migraine comes on suddenly. The head and neck muscles, reacting from continuous stress, become overworked. The tight muscles squeeze the arteries and reduce the blood flow. Then, when the person relaxes suddenly, the constricted muscles expand, stretching the blood vessel walls. With each heart beat, the blood pushes through these vessels and expands them further, causing intense pain.

Causes and Symptoms

There is a definite pattern of a migraine. The pain is on only one side of the head and often radiates from the eye. The right side of the head may be affected in one attack and the next time, the concentration of pain may be on the left side. Migraine attacks are usually preceded by a short period of depression, irritability, and loss of appetite. Some persons get attacks daily; others, every month or every two or three months; and still others, only once or twice in several years.

The main symptoms of migraine are a pounding pain, nausea, and vomiting. The blood vessels on the affected side of the head become prominent and pulsating. A migraine gives a fair warning before striking. The patient sees flashes of light or black spots or only parts of the objects in front of him. He may also feel

160

numbness or weakness in an arm or leg, or on one side of the face. Sometimes the numbness may affect both sides of the face, tongue, and the entire mouth, making the speech slurred and difficult. As the headache develops, disturbed digestion becomes a marked feature.

Migraine may result from a variety of causes such as low blood sugar, allergy, infection, excessive intake of certain drugs, a weak constitution, low energy, nutritional deficiency, consistent overwork, improper sleep and rest, excessive smoking, drinking, and sexual indulgence. Menstruation in women is also one of the important causes of migraine. This form of migraine usually abates after menopause.

Remedies

Grapes: The juice of ripe grapes is an effective home remedy for a migraine. It is said that King Jamshed of Persia, who was very fond of grapes, once stored the juice of grapes well packed in bottles and made it public that the bottles contained strong poison, so as to prevent others from taking it. It so happened that the king's wife was struck with migraine and having obtained no relief from any treatment, decided to end her life by taking this so-called 'poison'. She took it several times in small doses and contrary to her expectations, it gave her great relief instead of killing her.

Niacin: Niacin has proved helpful in the treatment of migraine. Valuable sources of this vitamin are yeast, whole wheat, green leafy vegetables, tomatoes, nuts, sunflower seeds, liver, and fish. Vitamin B complex tablets containing 100 mg of niacin can be taken for the same purpose.

Cabbage Leaf Compress: An ancient folk remedy for easing the pain of migraine is a cabbage leaf compress. A few leaves of the vegetable should be crushed, and then placed in a cloth and bound on the forehead at bedtime, or when convenient during the day. The compress should be renewed when the leaves dry out.

Lemon Crust: The crusts of lemon have also been found beneficial in the treatment of migraine. These crusts should be pounded into a fine paste in a mortar. The paste should be applied as a plaster on the forehead. It will provide great relief.

Vegetable Juices: Carrot juice, in combination with spinach juice, or beet and cucumber juices, has been found beneficial in the treatment of migraine. In the first combination, 200 ml of spinach juice may be mixed with 300 ml of carrot juice to prepare 500 ml or half a litre of the combined juices. In the second combination, 100 ml each of beet and cucumber juices may be mixed with 300 ml of carrot juice.

Dietary Considerations

It is essential to undertake a thorough cleansing of the system and adopt vitality-building measures. To begin with, the patient should resort to fasting on orange juice and water for two or three days. If the orange juice does not agree with the patient, juices of vegetables such as carrots, cucumber, and celery may be taken. After the short juice fast, the patient may adopt an all-fruit diet for about five days, taking three meals a day of fresh juicy fruits. Thereafter the patient should follow a well-balanced diet consisting of seeds, nuts, grains, vegetables, and fruits. This diet should be supplemented with milk, yoghurt, buttermilk, vegetable oils, and honey. Further short periods of the all-fruit diet may be necessary at intervals of a month or two, according to the requirement of the case.

Foods which should be avoided are white flour products, sugar, confectionery, rich cakes, pastries, sweets, refined cereals, greasy foods, tinned or preserved foods, pickles, condiments, and sauces. The patient should eat frequent small meals rather than a few large ones. Overeating should be avoided. Copious drinking of water is recommended.

Other Measures

During the initial two or three days of the juice fast, a warm-water enema may be taken daily to cleanse the bowels. A hot foot bath, fomentation over the stomach and spine, cold compresses (4.5^0C to 15.6^0C) applied to the head, and towels wrung out of very hot water and frequently applied to the neck will go a long way in relieving migraine headaches. The patient should also take plenty of exercise and walk in the fresh air.

Mumps

Inflammation of Parotid Glands

Mumps refer to a virus infection of the salivary glands, gonads, and, occasionally, other parts of the body. It is an infectious disease that occurs most frequently in children and young persons between the ages of five and fifteen years. Most persons have mumps only once in their lives, but one person in ten may have a second attack.

Causes and Symptoms

In children, the first sign of mumps is swelling of the salivary glands, but adults sometimes run a temperature and feel ill a couple of days before the glands enlarge. At first, the swelling is often uncomfortable or painful. If the disease occurs after puberty, the testicles may become swollen and painful in males; a similar condition may affect the female ovaries, sometimes leading to sterility.

Mumps is caused by a virus which attacks the salivary glands, particularly the parotid glands located on each side of the face just below and in front of the ear. The incubation period of the disease is about two weeks. Dietetic errors are at the root of the trouble.

Remedies

Chebulic Myroblan: Chebulic myroblan is one of the most effective remedies for mumps. A thick paste should be made from this herb by rubbing it in water. If applied over the swelling, it will provide relief.

Peepal Leaves: The leaves of the peepal tree are another effective home remedy for this disease. These leaves should be smeared with *ghee* and warmed over a fire. They should then be bandaged over the inflamed part for beneficial results.

Indian Aloe: The use of the herb Indian aloe is a well-known remedy in the indigenous system of medicine for any inflamed and painful part of the body. A piece of a leaf of this herb should be peeled on one side, warmed and then sprinkled with a little turmeric *(haldi)* and the extract of Indian barbery *(rasaut),* and then bandaged over the swelling.

Asparagus: The seeds of asparagus are valuable in mumps. These seeds, combined with an equal proportion of fenugreek *(methi)* seeds, should be ground together to the consistency of a paste. This paste can be applied over the swellings.

Ginger: Dry ginger is considered beneficial in the treatment of mumps. It should be made into a paste and applied over the swollen parts. As the paste dries, the swelling will be reduced and the pain will also subside.

Margosa Leaves: The leaves of margosa are also useful in the treatment of mumps. The leaves of this tree, combined with turmeric *(haldi)* should be made into a paste and applied externally over the affected parts. This will bring good results.

Dietary Considerations

To begin with, the patient should be kept on a diet of orange juice diluted with warm water on a 50:50 basis, for a few days. If the orange juice does not suit the patient, the juices of other fruits such as lemon *(mossambi),* apple, pineapple, grapes; or vegetables like carrots should be given.

When the patient can swallow food comfortably and the swelling has subsided, an all-fruit diet should be adopted for a day or two. Thereafter, he may be allowed to gradually embark upon a well-balanced diet of natural foods, with emphasis on fresh fruits and raw vegetables.

Other Measures

A warm-water enema should be used daily during the juice fast. Hot and cold fomentations should be applied every two hours during the day for about ten minutes, and should consist of two or three hot applications, followed by a cold one.

Nephritis

Inflammation of Kidneys

Nephritis refers to an inflammation of the kidneys. It is a serious condition and may be either acute or chronic. Most often this disease strikes in childhood or adolescence. It can become progressively worse and result in death, if not treated properly at the initial stage.

Causes and Symptoms

The main symptoms of acute nephritis are pain in the kidneys, extending down to the ureter, fever, dull pain in the back, and scanty and highly coloured urine. Often, the urine may contain blood, albumin, and casts consisting of clumps of red and white cells. Other symptoms are puffiness in the face, and swelling of the feet and ankles. In the chronic stages, the patient passes large amounts of albumin in the urine. Later, there may be a rise in blood pressure and the patient may develop uraemia.

Nephritis usually follows some streptococcus infection of the throat, or an attack of scarlet fever, or rheumatic fever. The underlying causes of this disease are, however, wrong feeding habits and weak defence mechanisms of the body.

Remedies

Carrot Juice: The use of carrot juice is one of the most effective home remedies for nephritis. One glass of carrot juice, mixed with a tablespoon of honey and a teaspoon of fresh lime juice, should be taken every day, first thing in the morning.

Banana: Bananas are an effective remedy for nephritis due to their low protein and salt, and high carbohydrate content. A diet of bananas only should be taken for three or four days, consuming eight to nine bananas a day in the treatment of this disease.

Avocado: Avocados are valuable as a staple food in nephritis. The usefulness of this fruit arises from its large mineral and small protein contents.

Grapes: Grapes are an excellent remedy for acute and chronic nephritis. They possess an exceptional diuretic value on account of their high contents of water and potassium salt. Their value in kidney troubles like nephritis is enhanced by their low albumin and sodium chloride content.

Coconut Water: Tender coconut water is another excellent remedy for this disease. The water of one green tender coconut can be taken beneficially once or twice a day. It acts as a very effective but safe diuretic in the treatment of nephritis.

Dietary Considerations

The safest treatment for acute nephritis is fasting on vegetable juices for seven to ten days. This will remove the toxins and systemic impurities responsible for the inflammatory kidney conditions. After the juice fast, the patient may adopt an all-fruit diet for four or five days. Thereafter, he may adopt a diet of fruits and milk for about a week, and then gradually adopt a well-balanced, low-protein vegetarian diet, with emphasis on fresh fruits, and raw and steamed vegetables.

In case of chronic nephritis, a short juice fast for three days may be followed by a restricted diet for ten days. Under this regimen, oranges or orange juice may be taken for breakfast. Lunch may consist of salad made of raw vegetables in season, and dinner may consist of one or two vegetables, steamed in their own juices, and a few nuts. Thereafter, the patient may gradually adopt a well-balanced, low-protein vegetarian diet.

Further juice fasts of short duration and a restricted diet for a week should be undertaken at intervals of two or three months until such time as the kidney condition shows signs of normalisation. The patient should avoid vegetables containing large quantities of oxalic acid, such as spinach and rhubarb. Chocolate and cocoa contain oxalic acid and must not be taken. Common salt should be eliminated from the diet. Five or six small meals should be taken in preference to a few large ones.

Other Measures

A warm-water enema should be taken each day to cleanse the bowels during the initial juice fast.

Neuritis

Inflammation of the Nerves

Neuritis refers to an inflammation of the nerves, be it a single nerve or a series of nerves. At times, several different groups of nerves in various parts of the body may be involved. This condition is known as polyneuritis.

Causes and Symptoms

The main symptoms of neuritis are a tingling and burning sensation, and stabbing pains in the affected nerves. In severe cases, there may be numbness, loss of sensation, and paralysis of the nearby muscles. Thus temporary paralysis of the face muscles may result from changes in the facial nerve on the affected side. During the acute stage of this condition, the patient may not be able to close his eyes due to a loss of normal tone and strength of the muscles on the affected side of the face.

The chief cause of neuritis is the presence of toxins in the blood and other body fluids. This could be the result of a faulty diet, wrong habits of living, overwork, nutritional deficiencies, and metabolic disturbances. Other causes include a blow or a penetrating injury; a bad bruise or heavy pressure over a nerve trunk; dislocation and fractures of the bones; certain infections; diabetes mellitus; and poisoning with insecticides, mercury, lead, arsenic, and alcohol.

Remedies

Soya Bean Milk: The most important among the home remedies in the treatment of neuritis is soya bean milk. A cup of this milk, mixed with a teaspoon of honey, should be taken every night. It tones up the nervous system due to its rich concentration of lecithin, vitamin B_1, and glutamic acid. Soya bean milk is prepared by soaking the beans in water for about twelve hours. The skin of the beans is then removed and after a thorough wash, they are turned into a fine paste in a grinding machine. The paste is mixed with water, three times its quantity. The milk is then boiled on a slow fire, and stirred frequently. After it becomes a little cooler, it should be strained through a cheese cloth and sugar added to it.

Barley Brew: Barley brew is another effective remedy for neuritis. It is prepared by boiling quarter of a cup of pearled barley grain in half a cup of water. When the water has boiled down to about one-quarter, it should be strained carefully. For better results, it should be mixed with half a glass of buttermilk and the juice of half a lime.

Carrot and Spinach: Raw carrots and spinach have proved valuable in neuritis as both these vegetables are rich in elements, the deficiency of which leads to this disease. The quickest and most effective way in which the body can obtain and assimilate these elements is by drinking at least half a litre of the combined raw juices of carrot and spinach — 300 ml of carrot juice and 200 ml of spinach juice — daily.

Orange Flowers: The use of orange flowers has also been found useful in neuritis. The water distilled from these flowers is a stimulating and refreshing drink, and should be taken regularly by the patient. The finest quality is one distilled from the petals of the bitter orange. Eating fresh orange flowers with honey is also an effective tonic for the nerves and valuable in treating neuritis, and about ten grams should be eaten daily.

Vitamin B: All vitamins of the B group are valuable in neuritis. A combination of vitamins B_1, B_2, B_6, B_{12}, and pantothenic acid have proved to be of immense help in this disease; in fact, extreme pain, weakness, and numbness, in some cases, have been relieved within an hour.

Dietary Considerations

The best treatment for neuritis is optimum nutrition, well assimilated with all the vitamins and other nutrients. The emphasis should be on whole grains, particularly, whole wheat, brown rice, raw and sprouted seeds, milk, yoghurt, and home-made cottage cheese. In severe cases, the patient should be put on a short juice fast for four or five days before being given the optimum diet. Carrots, beet, citrus fruits, apples, and pineapples may be used for juices. The patient should avoid white bread, sugar, refined cereals, meat, fish, tinned foods, tea, coffee, and condiments.

Other Measures

The patient should be given two or three hot baths with Epsom salts weekly. He should remain in the bath for twenty-five to thirty minutes. The affected parts should also be bathed several times daily in hot water containing Epsom salts — a tablespoon of salt to a cup of hot water. Walking and other moderate exercises are also beneficial in the treatment of neuritis.

Obesity

Overweight

Obesity may be described as a condition characterised by excessive deposition or storage of fat in the body. It usually results from consumption of food in excess of physiological needs. Obesity is common among people in Western countries and among the higher income groups in India and other developing countries.

Causes and Symptoms

Obesity is a serious health hazard as the extra fat puts a strain on the heart, kidneys, and liver as well as the large weight-bearing joints such as the hips, knees, and ankles, all of which shortens the life span. It has been truly said: 'The longer the belt, the shorter the life'. Overweight persons are susceptible to several diseases like coronary thrombosis, heart failure, high blood pressure, diabetes, arthritis, gout, liver, and gall-bladder disorders.

Most often, the chief cause of obesity is overeating, that is, the intake of calories beyond the body's energy requirement. Some people have a habit of consuming high-calorie foods. Obesity is rarely the result of disturbances of the thyroid or pituitary glands. Glandular disorders account for only about two per cent of the total incidence.

Remedies

Lime Juice-Honey: Fasting on lime juice-honey water is highly beneficial in the treatment of obesity. In this mode of treatment, one teaspoon of fresh honey should be mixed with the juice of half a lime in a glass of lukewarm water and taken at regular intervals.

Lemon Juice: Another effective remedy for obesity is an exclusive lemon juice diet. On the first day, the patient should be given nothing but plenty of water. On the second day, the diet should consist of the juice of three lemons, mixed with an equal amount of water. Subsequently, one lemon should be increased each day until the juice of twelve lemons is consumed per day. Then the number of lemons should be decreased in the same order until three lemons are taken in a day. The patient may feel weak and hungry on the first two days, but afterwards, his condition will stabilise.

Jujube: The leaves of jujube or Indian plum are another valuable remedy for obesity. A handful of leaves should be soaked overnight in water and this water should be taken in the morning, preferably on an empty stomach. This treatment should be continued for at least one month to achieve beneficial results.

Cabbage: Cabbage is considered to be an excellent home remedy for obesity. Recent research has revealed that a valuable chemical called tartaric acid is present in this vegetable which inhibits the conversion of sugar and other carbohydrates into fat. Hence, it is of great value in weight reduction. Substituting a meal with cabbage salad would be the simplest way to stay slim.

Tomato: Tomatoes are valuable in obesity. One or two ripe tomatoes taken early morning as a substitute for breakfast, for a couple of months, are considered a safe method of weight reduction. They also supply the food elements essential to preserve health.

Finger Millet: Finger millet is an ideal food for the obese, because its digestion is slow and due to this, the carbohydrates take a longer time to get absorbed. By eating preparations made of ragi, the constant desire to eat is curbed, thus reducing the daily calorie intake. At the same time, ragi supplies an abundant quantity of calcium, phosphorus, iron, vitamin B_1 and B_2, and prevents malnutrition in spite of restricted food.

Dietary Considerations

To begin with, the patient should undertake a juice fast for seven to ten days. Juices of lemon, grapefruit, orange, pineapple, cabbage, and celery may be taken during this period. After the juice fast, the patient should spend four or five days on an all-fruit diet, taking three meals of fresh juicy fruits daily. Thereafter, he may gradually embark upon a low-calorie, well-balanced diet of seeds, nuts, grains, vegetables, and fruits, with emphasis on raw fruits, vegetables, and fresh juices.

The foods which should be drastically curtailed or altogether avoided are high-fat foods such as butter, cheese, chocolate, cream, ice cream, fat meats, fried foods and gravies; high-carbohydrate foods like breads, candy, cake, cookies, cereal products, legumes, potatoes, sugar, syrup and rich puddings; beverages such as all soft drinks; and alcoholic drinks.

Other Measures

The patient should adopt all other natural methods of reducing weight. These include exercise such as walking, swimming, bicycling; yogic *asanas,* and deep breathing exercises; and measures to bring on excessive perspiration such as sauna baths, steam baths, and heavy massage. Above all, obese persons should make every effort to avoid negative emotions such as anxiety, fear, hostility, and insecurity, and develop a positive outlook on life.

Palpitation

Irregular Heartbeat

Palpitation, a common problem, is a state in which the heart beats forcibly and, maybe, irregularly. It enables the person to become aware of the action of his heart. It is a distressing condition but is not always serious.

Causes and Symptoms

The main symptom of palpitation of the heart is a kind of 'thumping' feeling in the chest. The patient feels a real discomfort in the front of the chest. The pulse rate may become faster than normal.

Palpitation of the heart may occur due to a variety of factors, most of which may not be related to the heart itself. Anything which increases the work load of the heart may bring on this condition. Some persons may experience palpitations when lying on the left side, because the heart is nearer the chest wall in that position. Many nervous persons suffer from this condition. Although palpitations do occur among other symptoms in serious heart disease, the vast majority of cases are due to anxiety and have no direct connection with heart disease whatsoever. Other causes contributing to this condition are an overful stomach, flatulence, and constipation. Excessive smoking may also give rise to this disorder.

Remedies

Grapes: Grapes are one of the most effective home remedies for palpitation of the heart. The patient should take the juice of this fruit at frequent intervals. This will relieve the condition.

Guava: The use of guava is another effective home remedy for palpitation of the heart. The patient should eat a ripe guava daily on an empty stomach. It is especially beneficial if this disorder caused by nervousness and anaemia.

Snake Gourd Leaves: The leaves of snake gourd have been found beneficial in the treatment of palpitation of the heart. The juice of these leaves should be extracted and given in doses of one to two tablespoons thrice daily.

Honey: Honey has proved valuable in overcoming this condition. Honey is considered to be an excellent food for the heart, being easily digested and assimilated. The patient should take a glass of water, mixed with a tablespoon of honey and the juice of half a lemon, before going to bed.

Indian Spikenard: The herb Indian spikenard is also beneficial in the treatment of palpitation of the heart. It stimulates the action of the heart. It should be taken in doses of two to three grams with the addition of a pinch of camphor and cinnamon. It can also be taken as an infusion in doses of 30 to 60 ml, three times a day.

Aniseed and Dry Coriander: A mixture of powdered aniseed, dry coriander, and jaggery can also be used beneficially in the treatment of this condition. Equal quantities of each of these three substances should be powdered. About six grams of this mixed powder should be taken after each meal by the patient suffering from palpitation of the heart.

Dietary Considerations

The patient suffering from palpitation of the heart should take a simple diet of natural foods, with emphasis on fresh fruits, and raw or lightly cooked vegetables. He should avoid tea, coffee, alcohol, chocolate, soft drinks, all white flour products, sugar, food colourings, chemical additives, white rice, and strong condiments. He should restrict his diet to three meals a day. He should take fruits, milk, and a handful of nuts or seeds for breakfast in the morning; steamed vegetables, wholewheat *chapatis* and a glass of buttermilk for lunch in the afternoon; and fresh green vegetable salad, sprouts of alfalfa seeds and *mung,* and cottage cheese or a glass of buttermilk for dinner.

Other Measures

The patient must learn the art of meditation and relaxation. *Shavasana* is ideal for this purpose. The patient should also undertake some form of active exercise such as brisk walks, swimming, skipping, and cycling.

Peptic Ulcer

Stomach Ulcer

A peptic ulcer refers to an eroded lesion in the inner lining of the stomach and the adjoining intestinal tract called the duodenum. The ulcer located in the stomach is known as a gastric ulcer, and that located in the duodenum is called a duodenal ulcer. Usually, both are grouped together and termed as peptic ulcer.

Causes and Symptoms

The symptoms of peptic ulcer are sharp and severe pain and

discomfort in the upper part of the abdomen. Gastric ulcer pain usually occurs an hour after meals and rarely at night. Duodenal ulcer pain usually occurs between meals when the stomach is empty. The pain is relieved by food, especially milk. As the disease progresses, there is distension of the stomach due to excessive flatulence, mental tension, insomnia, and gradual weakening of the body. Blood may also be detected in the stool.

A peptic ulcer is the result of hyperacidity, which is caused by an increase in the hydrochloric acid in the stomach. This strong acid, secreted by the cells lining the stomach, erodes the inner lining of the stomach. Dietetic indiscretion such as overeating, taking of heavy meals or highly spiced foods, coffee, alcohol, and smoking are the main factors contributing to this condition. Other causes are the ingestion of certain drugs, food poisoning, certain infections, gout, emotional disturbances, stress, and nervous tension.

Remedies

Banana: Banana is one of the most effective home remedies for the treatment of a peptic ulcer. This fruit is said to contain an unidentified compound, perhaps jokingly called vitamin U (against ulcers). Banana neutralises the over-acidity of the gastric juices and reduces the irritation of the ulcer by coating the lining of the stomach. Patients who are in an advanced state of the disease should take a diet consisting only of two bananas with a glass of milk, three or four times a day.

Wood Apple: An infusion of the leaves of wood apple is another effective remedy for this disease. Fifteen grams of leaves should be soaked overnight in 250 ml of water. In the morning this water should be strained and taken as a drink. The pain and discomfort will be relieved when this treatment is continued for a few weeks. *Bael* leaves are rich in tannins which reduce inflammation and help in the healing of ulcers. The *bael* fruit taken in the form of a beverage also has great healing properties on account of its mucilage content. This substance forms a coating on the stomach mucosa and thus helps in the healing of ulcers.

Lime: Lime is valuable in peptic ulcers. The citric acid in this fruit, together with the mineral salts present in the juice, help in digestion.

Cabbage: Cabbage is regarded as another useful home remedy for a peptic ulcer: 250 gm should be boiled in 500 ml of water till it is reduced to half; this water should be allowed to cool, and taken twice daily. The juice extracted from raw cabbage is also a valuable medicine for a peptic ulcer. However, as this juice is very strong, it should be taken in combination with carrot juice, in quantities of 125 ml each.

Fenugreek Seeds: A tea made from fenugreek seeds is yet another useful remedy for peptic ulcers. The seeds, when moistened with water, are slightly mucilaginous. The tea helps in the healing of ulcers as the mild coating of mucilaginous material deposited by fenugreek, passes through the stomach and intestines, providing protective shell for the ulcers.

Drumstick: The leaves of the *kalyana murangal* tree, which is a variety of drumstick found in South India, have also proved helpful in the healing of ulcers. Ten grams of the leaves of this tree should be ground into a paste, mixed with half a cup of yoghurt, and taken daily.

Vegetable Juices: The juices of raw vegetables, particularly carrot and cabbage, are beneficial in the treatment of peptic ulcers. Carrot juice may be taken either alone or in combination with spinach, or beet and cucumber. The formula proportions in case of the first combination are 300 ml of carrot juice and 200 ml of spinach juice; and in case of the second combination, 300 ml of carrot juice and 100 ml each of beet and cucumber juice to make 500 ml of juice.

Almond Milk: Milk prepared from blanched almonds in a blender is very useful as a treatment for peptic ulcers. It binds the excess of acid in the stomach and supplies high quality protein.

Goat's Milk: Goat's milk is also highly beneficial in the treatment of this disease. It actually helps to heal peptic ulcers. For better results, a glass of goat's milk should be taken in a raw state, three times daily.

Dietary Considerations

The diet of the patient suffering from a peptic ulcer should be so planned as to provide adequate nutrition, while affording rest to the disturbed organs, maintaining continuous neutralisation of the gastric acid, inhibiting the production of acid, and reducing mechanical and chemical irritation. Milk, cream, butter, fruits, fresh raw and boiled vegetables, natural foods, and natural vitamin supplements constitute the best diet.

Other Measures

A daily massage and deep breathing exercises also help. Above all, the patient must try to rid himself of worries and stay cheerful. He should also cultivate regularity in his habits — be it work, exercise, or rest. Yogic *asanas* which are beneficial in the treatment of hyperacidity and ulcers are *vajrasana, uttanpadasana, pavanmuktasana, bhujangasana,* and *paschimottanasana.*

Piles

Haemorrhoids

Piles or haemorrhoids is one of the most common ailments today. It is a varicose and often inflamed condition of the veins, inside or just outside the rectum. In external piles, there is a lot of pain but not much bleeding. In the case of internal piles, there is discharge of dark blood. In some cases the veins burst and this results in what is known as bleeding piles.

Causes and Symptoms

Pain at passing stools, slight bleeding in the case of internal trouble, and feeling of soreness and irritation after passing a stool are the usual symptoms of piles. The pat ent cannot sit comfortably due to itching, discomfort, and pain in the rectal region.

The primary cause of piles is chronic constipation and other bowel disorders. The straining in order to evacuate the constipated bowels, and the pressure thus caused on the surrounding veins leads to piles. Piles are more common during pregnancy and in conditions affecting the liver and upper bowel. Other causes are prolonged periods of standing or sitting, strenuous work, obesity, general weakness of the tissues of the body, mental tension, and heredity.

Remedies

Dry Figs: The use of dry figs is one of the most effective home remedies for piles. Three or four figs should be soaked overnight in water after being cleaned thoroughly in hot water. They should be taken first thing in the morning along with the water in which they were soaked. They should also be taken in the evening in a similar manner. This treatment should be continued for three or four weeks. The tiny seeds of the fruit possess an excellent quality of stimulating peristaltic movements of the intestines. This facilitates easy evacuation of faeces and keeps the alimentary canal clean. The pressure on the anus thus being relieved, the hemorrhoids also contract.

Mango Seeds: Mango seeds are an effective remedy for bleeding piles. The seeds should be collected during the mango season, dried in the shade, powdered, and kept stored for use as medicine. This powder should be given in doses of about one and a half to two grams with or without honey, twice daily.

Jambul Fruit: The jambul fruit is another effective remedy for bleeding piles. The fruit should be taken with salt every morning for two or three months during its season. The use of the fruit in this manner during every season will effect a complete cure and save the user from bleeding piles for his entire life.

Radish: White radish is considered highly valuable in piles; 100 mg of grated radish mixed with a teaspoon of honey may be taken twice daily in treating this condition. This vegetable can also be taken in the form of juice mixed with a pinch of salt. It should be given in doses of 60 to 90 ml, morning and evening. White radish, well ground into a paste in milk, can also be applied over inflamed pile masses to relieve pain and swelling.

Turnip: The leaves of turnip have been found useful in this disease. The juice of these leaves should be extracted and 150 ml given to the patient. It is, however, necessary to take a proper diet of raw fruits and vegetables while taking this juice. For better results, 50 ml of the juice should be mixed with equal quantities of juices of watercress, spinach, and carrots.

Bitter Gourd: The juice of the fresh leaves of bitter gourd is also valuable in piles. Three teaspoons of the leaf juice, mixed with a glass of buttermilk, should be taken every morning for treating this condition. A paste of the roots of the bitter gourd plant can also be applied over piles with beneficial results.

Ginger: Ginger is also useful in this disease. Half a teaspoon of fresh ginger juice, mixed with one teaspoon each of fresh lime juice and fresh mint juice, and a tablespoon of honey, constitutes an effective medicine for piles.

Onion: Onions are valuable in bleeding piles. About thirty grams of this vegetable should be finely rubbed in water and sixty grams of sugar added to it. It should be taken twice daily by the patient. It will bring relief within a few days. Onion is also useful in the treatment of dry piles. A crushed onion, skinned and roasted in aches, may be applied with beneficial results.

Rice: Rice has a very low fibre content and is, therefore, extremely soothing to the digestive system. A thick gruel of rice, mixed with a glass of buttermilk and a ripe banana, given twice a day, is a very nutritious diet for a patient with piles.

Wheat Grass: Wheat grass juice used as an enema helps detoxify the walls of the piles. The general procedure is to give an enema with lukewarm or *neem* water. After waiting for twenty minutes, 90 to 120 ml of the wheat grass juice enema is given. This should be retained for fifteen minutes.

Sesame Seeds: Sesame seeds are also valuable in piles. They can be taken in the form of a decoction by boiling twenty grams of seeds in 500 ml of water till it is reduced by one-third, or as sweetmeats. Ground to paste with water, they can be given with butter for bleeding piles.

Chebulic Myroblan: The herb chebulic myroblan is a popular remedy for piles. It is very effective as a laxative and is highly astringent. The fruit should be roasted to a brown colour in cluster oil, and then powdered and stored. Half a teaspoon of this powder at bedtime will bring about normal bowel movements in the morning, and the astringent property of the fruit will heal the pile masses. A decoction of the herb prepared by boiling six to seven dry fruits in half a litre of water should be used for washing bleeding piles. The paste of the fruit mixed in a bland oil is good as an external application.

Dietary Considerations

The treatment of the basic cause, namely, chronic constipation, is the only way to get rid of the trouble. To begin with, the entire digestive tract must be given a complete rest for a few days and the intestines thoroughly cleansed. For this purpose, the patient should adopt an all-fruit diet for, at least, seven days. Thereafter he may adopt a diet of natural foods aimed at securing soft stools.

Other Measures

A patient with piles must make an all-out effort to tone up the entire system. Exercise plays an important corrective role in this condition. Movements which exercise the abdominal muscles will improve circulation in the rectal region and relieve congestion.

Pneumonia

Pneumonia refers to the inflammation of the lungs. It is one of the most serious infectious diseases. The disease assumes alarming proportions if both the lungs are affected; this condition is called double pneumonia in common parlance.

Causes and Symptoms

Most cases of pneumonia begin with a cold in the head or throat. The patient generally feels a chill, shivering fever, difficulty in breathing, and sharp pain in the chest. This may be followed by a cough with pinkish sputum, which may later become brownish. In young children, the disease may cause delirium and convulsions. The temperature may rise to 40.6^0C and the pulse may go upto 150 beats per minute. A common complication of pneumonia is pleurisy.

Pneumonia is caused by various types of germs such as streptococcus, staphylococcus, and pneumococcus. At times, certain viruses are also responsible for this disease. Other causes are fungal infections, irritation by worms, inhaling foreign matter, irritant dust, or noxious gases. The real cause of pneumonia, however, is a constitution weakened by the presence of toxins in the body, especially in the lungs and air passages. The accumulation of toxins is due to wrong feeding habits and a faulty lifestyle.

Remedies

Fenugreek: During the early acute stage of pneumonia, a tea made from fenugreek seeds will help the body to produce perspiration, dispel toxicity, and shorten the period of fever. Upto four cups of the tea can be taken daily. The quantity can be reduced as the condition improves. To improve the flavour of the tea, a few drops of lemon juice may be added. During this treatment, no other food or nourishment should be taken, as fasting and fenugreek will allow the body to correct these respiratory problems in a few days.

Garlic: Garlic is a marvellous remedy for pneumonia, if given in sufficient quantities. It brings down the temperature, as well as the pulse and respiration within forty-eight hours. A paste of garlic can also be applied externally on the chest with beneficial results as it is an irritant and rubefacient.

Sesame Seeds: Sesame seeds are valuable in pneumonia. An infusion of the seeds can be made by steeping 15 gm of seeds in 250 ml of water. This infusion, mixed with a tablespoon of linseed, a pinch of common salt, and a dessertspoon of honey, should be given in the treatment of this disease. This will help remove catarrhal matter and phlegm from the bronchial tubes.

Parsnip Juice: The juice of parsnip, a root vegetable botanically known as *Pastinaca sativa,* has been found beneficial in the treatment of pneumonia. The juice of the leaves and root of this plant possess high therapeutic value. The phosphorus and chlorine elements contained therein are of particular benefit to the lungs and the bronchial system, thus making the juice an excellent home remedy for pneumonia. The patient should take 250 ml of juice daily. It is, however, essential that only the juice of the cultivated parsnip plant should be used for this purpose. The wild variety must not be used in juices as it contains some poisonous ingredients.

Other Vegetable Juices: The juice of carrots, in combination either with spinach juice, or beet and cucumber juices, has also been found useful in pneumonia. In these combinations, 200 ml of spinach juice or 100 ml each of beet and cucumber juices should be mixed with 300 ml of carrot juice to prepare 500 ml or half a litre of combined juice.

Turpentine Oil: The pain of pneumonia can be relieved by rubbing oil of turpentine over the rib cage and wrapping warmed cotton wool over it.

Dietary Considerations

At the beginning of the treatment, the patient should be kept on a diet of raw juices for five to ten days, depending on the severity of the disease. He should take a glass of fruit or vegetable juice, diluted with warm water, every two or three hours. After a diet of raw juices, when the fever subsides, the patient should spent three or four days on an exclusive fresh fruit diet, taking three meals a day of juicy fruits. Thereafter, he may gradually adopt a well-balanced diet of natural foods, with emphasis on fresh fruits and raw vegetables.

Other Measures

The patient should be given a warm-water enema daily to cleanse the bowels during the period of raw juice therapy and the all-fruit diet, and thereafter when necessary. To reduce temperature during the course of the fever, the procedure outlined in the chapter on Malaria (see pp. 150 to 152) should be followed.

Premature Greying of Hair

Loss of Black Pigment of Hair

The hair has a tendency to lose its natural colour with advancing age and turn grey, but premature greying is a morbid condition and it makes even the young look older.

The hair is an appendage of the skin. It is composed of the same kinds of cells as are found in the outer layer of the skin, which is known as the epidermis. Hair grows from hair follicles which are deep recesses in the epidermis. The sebaceous glands of the scalp secrete an oily substance called sebum, which is the source of nutrition, lustre, and blackness of the hair. The hair cannot be fed externally, for such nourishment, as the scalp requires, must come to it from the bloodstream.

Causes and Symptoms

A faulty diet and mental worries are the two primary causes of premature greying of hair. Lack of some of the B vitamins, iron, copper, and iodine in the daily diet is said to be a contributory factor. Mental worries produce extraordinary tension in the skin of the scalp; this interferes with the supply of vital nutrition necessary for the health of the hair. Other causes of premature greying of hair are an unclean condition of the scalp, washing the hair with hot water, drying it with an electric dryer, and use of hair dyes. Heredity is also a predisposing factor.

Remedies

Indian Gooseberry: The use of Indian gooseberry is the foremost among the home remedies found beneficial in the prevention and treatment of premature greying of hair. This is a valuable hair tonic for enriching hair growth and hair pigmentation. The fruit, cut into pieces, should be dried, preferably in the shade. These pieces should be boiled in coconut oil till the solid matter becomes like charred dust. This darkish oil is very useful against premature greying.

The water in which dried *amla* pieces have been soaked overnight is also nourishing for the hair. This water should be used for the last rinse while washing the hair. Massaging the scalp every night with a teaspoonful of *amla* juice, mixed with a teaspoon of almond oil and a few drops of lime juice, also proves beneficial in the prevention and treatment of premature greying of hair.

Amaranth: Amaranth is another effective home remedy for hair disorders. Application of the fresh juice of the leaves of this vegetable helps the hair to retain its black colour and prevents it from premature greyness. It also helps the growth of the hair and keeps it soft.

Curry Leaves: Liberal intake of curry leaves is considered beneficial in preventing premature greying of hair. These leaves have the property of providing vitality and strength to hair roots. New hair roots that grow are healthier and contain a normal pigment. The leaves can be used in the form of a *chutney,* or may be squeezed in buttermilk. When the leaves are boiled in coconut oil, the oil forms an excellent hair tonic to stimulate hair growth and bring back hair pigmentation.

Ribbed Gourd: Ribbed gourd boiled in coconut oil is also an effective remedy for premature greying of hair. Pieces of this vegetable should be dried in the shade. These dried pieces should be soaked in coconut oil and kept aside for three or four days. The oil should then be boiled till the solid is reduced to a blackened residue. This oil should be massaged into the scalp. It will help enrich the hair roots and restore pigment to the hair.

Butter: The butter made from cow's milk has the property of preventing premature greying of hair. A small roll may be taken internally and a little quantity may be massaged into the hair roots twice a week.

Vitamins: The vitamins considered useful in guarding against premature greying of hair are pantothenic acid, para-aminobenzoic acid (paba), inositol. The minimum daily requirement of these vitamins appears to be 10 mg of pantothenic acid, 100 mg of para-aminobenzoic acid, and 2 gm of inositol. To obtain satisfactory results, all three of these vitamins belonging to the B group should be supplied at one time, preferably in a form which supplies all the B vitamins, such as yeast and liver. The three anti-greying-hair vitamins can also be produced in the intestinal tract by bacteria. Thus, taking a sufficient quantity of yoghurt daily and a tablespoonful

181

of yeast before each meal is an excellent remedy for the prevention and treatment of premature greying of hair. If one wishes to take tablets of calcium pantothenate and para-aminobenzoic acid (paba), they should be taken in addition to the yeast and yoghurt, and not as a substitute for them.

Dietary Considerations

Diet is of utmost importance in the prevention and treatment of premature greying of hair and persons suffering from this disorder should take a diet rich in all essential nutrients. Devitalising foods such as white flour, refined sugar and all products made from them, soft drinks, pastries, jams and jellies should be avoided. These foods take away energy, cause wrinkles, unattractive skin, grey hair, and premature old age.

Other Measures

Massage of the scalp with almond oil is recommended.

Prostate Disorders

Enlarged Prostate, Prostatitis

A large percentage of men over fifty years of age suffer from prostate troubles of one form or other. The prostate gland is a male gland, comparable in shape and size to a large chestnut. It is situated at the base of the urinary bladder and around the commencement of the urethra. There are various types of prostate disorders, the more important being hypertrophy or enlargement of the prostate gland, and prostatitis or inflammation in the prostate gland.

Causes and Symptoms

There are two warning signals to indicate the possibility of prostate disorders. The first is the interference with the passage of urine, and the second is the need to void the urine frequently during the night's sleep. Other symptoms are a dull aching pain in the lower back and pain in the hips, legs, and feet.

The position of the prostate gland makes it liable to congestion and other disorders. In an erect position, pressure falls on the pelvic region just where the prostate gland is situated. With ageing, the body gets heavier and loses its flexibility. This puts greater pressure on the pelvis and increases the vulnerability of the prostate gland. Prolonged periods of sitting, as in certain occupations, also increase the pressure on the pelvic region, resulting in congestion of the tissues in and around the prostate gland. Acute prostatitis may also result from exposure to cold and chill, and from infectious diseases. Chronic prostatis is an after-effect of the acute condition. It may also be caused by continual irritation of the gland due to excessive sexual excitement. Another important cause of prostate disorders is constipation, when the faeces become hardened and the rectum or lower bowel is overloaded, causing undue pressure on the prostate gland.

Remedies

Pumpkin Seeds: Pumpkin seeds are an effective home remedy for prostate problems and many patients have been helped by their use. These seeds are rich in unsaturated fatty acids which are essential to the health of the prostate. Persons beyond the age of fifty, who have any signs of prostate trouble; or those who suffer from urinary disorders of some kind, namely, burning or difficulty in passing urine freely, should take sixty to ninety grams of pumpkin seeds per day. The seeds may be taken in the form of powder sprinkled over cooked vegetables or mixed with wheat flour to make *chapatis*. They can also be taken in the form of a paste made with honey, or as a drink mixed with diluted milk and sugar to taste.

Vegetable Juices: The use of vegetable juices has been found beneficial in the treatment of prostate problems, including prostate enlargement. The juice of carrots, taken separately in a 500 ml quantity, or in combination with spinach juice, is specially valuable. In the case of combined juices, 200 ml of spinach juice should be mixed with 300 ml of carrot juice to prepare 500 ml or half a litre of combined juices.

Zinc: The use of zinc has been found valuable in cases of prostate disorders. About thirty milligrams of this mineral should be taken daily in the treatment of these diseases.

Vitamin E: Vitamin E has proved to be an important factor for prostate health. The patient should therefore use vitamin E-rich foods liberally or take 600 IU of this vitamin daily. Vitamin E-rich foods are wholegrain products, green leafy vegetables, eggs, milk, and all raw or sprouted seeds.

Dietary Considerations

To begin with, the patient should forego all solid foods and subsist on water, mixed with a little lemon juice, for two or three days. The water may be taken cold or hot and it should be taken every hour or so during waking hours. This will greatly increase the flow of urine. After the short fast, the patient may adopt an all-fruit diet, consisting of juicy fruits, for the next three days. This should be followed by a diet consisting of two meals of fruits and one of cooked vegetables for seven days. Thereafter, the patient may adopt a well-balanced diet, with emphasis on seeds, nuts, grains, vegetables, and fruits. Heavy starches, sweet stimulants, and highly seasoned foods are entirely forbidden, as they are said to cause direct irritation to the prostate gland and bladder. The diet should also exclude spices, condiments, salt in excess, sauces, red meats, cheese, asparagus, watercress, greasy or fried foods, alcohol, tobacco, and too much of tea or coffee. The patient should avoid hurried meals and must chew his food thoroughly and slowly. Water should be taken between meals and not at meal times.

Other Measures

During the initial water fast for two to three days, an enema may be taken once a day to clear the lower bowel of accumulations.

Hot and cold applications are highly beneficial in the treatment of prostate disorders. After a thorough cleansing of the bowels through a warm-water enema, hot and cold applications may be used directly on the prostate gland and its surrounding parts. The heat will relieve the tissues and a brief cold immersion will tone them up. The patient should take alternate hot and cold hip baths. These are of great value in relieving pain and reducing congestion.

A wet girdle pack is another valuable remedy in the realm of hydrotherapy which provides great relief in prostatitis and prostate enlargement. For this mode of treatment, thin cotton underwear and thick or woollen underwear are required. The thin underwear should be wrung in cold water and worn by the patient. The thick dry underwear should be worn above the wet underwear. This treatment should be continued for ninety minutes regularly every night. If the patient feels chilly, he should be covered with a blanket.

The patient should avoid sexual excess, irregularities in eating and drinking, long periods of sitting, and vigorous exercise. All efforts should be made to tone up the general condition of the body.

Psoriasis

Psoriasis is one of the most stubborn skin diseases. It is a chronic disease, characterised by thick, red, silvery, scaled patches of the skin. This disease affects both sexes equally, and is more common during the first fifteen to thirty years, although it may appear at any age. Psoriasis is not contagious.

Causes and Symptoms

Generally, the skin of the person suffering from this disease appears red and irritated and may be covered with bright silvery scales. Sometimes there is also a little itching. The areas usually involved are the elbows, knees, the skin behind the ears, the trunk, and the scalp. The disease may also affect the underarms and genital areas. The lesions vary in size from minute papules to sheets covering large parts of the body. Quite often, they are discs from half an inch to several inches in size. The lesions are always dry and rarely become infected.

Recent studies have shown that psoriasis involves an abnormality in the mechanism in which the skin grows and replaces itself. The abnormality is related to the metabolism of amino acids, the nature's basic building blocks for the reproduction of cell tissues. Heredity also plays a role in the development of psoriasis as it tends to occur in families. The factors that aggravate and precipitate the outbreak of this disease are physical and emotional stress, infections, and use of certain medicines for the treatment of other diseases.

Remedies

Cabbage Leaves: Cabbage leaves have been successfully used in the form of compresses in the treatment of psoriasis. The thickest and greenest outer leaves are most effective for use as compresses. They should be thoroughly washed in warm water and dried with a towel. The leaves should be flattened, softened and smoothed out by rolling them with a rolling pin after removing the thick veins. They should be warmed and then applied smoothly to the affected part in an overlapping manner. A pad of soft woollen cloth should be put over them. The whole compress should then be secured with an elastic bandage.

Bitter Gourd: Bitter gourd is a valuable remedy for psoriasis. A cup of fresh juice of this vegetable, mixed with a teaspoon of lime juice, should be taken sip by sip, on an empty stomach daily for four to six months.

Avocado Oil: The oil of avocado has been found beneficial in the treatment of this disease. It should be applied gently to the affected parts.

Cashewnut Oil: The oil extracted from the outer shell of the cashewnut is acrid and rubefacient. It can be applied beneficially on the affected area.

Buttermilk: The use of curd in the form of buttermilk has proved useful in psoriasis and the patient should drink it in liberal quantities. The application of buttermilk compresses over the affected parts will also be useful in treating this condition.

Vitamin E: Vitamin E therapy has been found effective in the treatment of psoriasis. The patient should take this vitamin in therapeutic doses of 400 mg a day. It will help reduce itching and scab formation.

Lecithin: Lecithin is also considered a remarkable remedy for psoriasis. The patient may take six to nine lecithin capsules a day—two or three capsules before or after each meal. If taken in the form of granules, four tablespoonfuls may be taken daily for two months. The dosage may be reduced thereafter to two tablespoons.

Dietary Considerations

Since psoriasis is a metabolic disease, a cleansing juice fast for a week is always desirable at the beginning of the treatment. Carrots, beets, cucumbers, and grapes may be used for juices. After the juice fast, the patient should adopt a well-balanced diet, consisting of seeds, nuts, grains, vegetables, and fruits. Emphasis should be placed on raw seeds and nuts, especially sesame seeds, pumpkin seeds, sunflower seeds, and plenty of organically grown raw vegetables and fruits. All animal fats, including milk, butter, eggs; refined or processed foods; foods containing hydrogenated fats or white sugar; all condiments; and tea and coffee should be avoided. When there is a substantial improvement, goat's milk, yoghurt, and home-made cottage cheese may be added to the diet. The juice fast may be repeated after a month or so.

Other Measures

During the initial juice fast, a warm-water enema should be used daily to cleanse the bowels. Frequent baths should be avoided. Soap should not be used. Regular sea-water baths and application of sea water externally over the affected parts once a day are beneficial. Hot Epsom salts baths also prove valuable in psoriasis. After an Epsom salts bath, a little olive oil may be applied. The skin should be kept absolutely clean by dry friction or daily sponging.

Pyorrhoea

Pus in the Gums

Pyorrhoea, or periodontal disease, to give it a proper medical term, is a disease of the gums. It is one of the most widely prevalent diseases. It affects the membrane surrounding the roots of the teeth and leads to loosening of the teeth, pus formation, and shrinkage of the gum. This disease is the primary cause for tooth loss among adults.

Causes and Symptoms

The gums become tender, and on pressing, pus oozes out along the margin of the teeth. Pus from the cavities continually finds its way into the stomach. When the disease is far advanced, the gums become swollen, and the stomach, being dosed with increasing quantities of pus, does not function properly. A sepsis may appear in various forms; digestion gets disturbed, liver trouble sets in, and the whole system is adversely affected.

Pyorrhoea is triggered by bacterial activity. A thin layer of harmful bacteria is continuously building up on our teeth. If it is not removed by tooth-cleansing, especially after meals, it forms an organised mass on the tooth surface in a short time. This is referred to as a 'bacterial plaque'. When accumulated, bacteria in plaque produce many toxins which irritate the gums, causing them to become inflamed, tender, and prone to bleeding easily. The bacterial activity is, however, facilitated by the lowered vitality of the system. Other factors contributing to the development of pyorrhoea include injury to the gums and supporting structures by physical and chemical irritants in the mouth, incorrect brushing, stagnation of food particles, and improper use of tooth picks.

Remedies

Guava: Chewing unripe guava is an excellent tonic for the teeth and gums. It stops the bleeding from the gums due to its styptic effect and richness in vitamin C. Chewing the tender leaves of the guava tree also helps in curing bleeding from the gums and keeps the teeth healthy. A decoction of root-bark can also be beneficially used as a mouthwash for swollen gums.

Lemon and Lime: The regular use of lemon and lime is useful in pyorrhoea due to their high vitamin C content. They strengthen the gums and teeth, and are very effective in preventing and curing acute inflammations of the gum margins.

Orange: The use of orange has also been found beneficial in the treatment of pyorrhoea. This fruit should be eaten regularly and its skin rubbed over the teeth and gums. This will improve the condition.

Pomegranate Rind: Powder of the dry rind of pomegranate, mixed with pepper and common salt, can be applied as a very good dentifrice. Its regular application strengthens the gums, stops bleeding, and prevents pyorrhoea.

Spinach Juice: The juice of raw spinach is another valuable remedy for the prevention and treatment of pyorrhoea because of its beneficial effect on the teeth and gums. This effect is greatly enhanced if spinach juice is taken in combination with carrot juice. Both spinach juice and carrot juice should be taken in quantities of 125 ml each daily. A permanent aid for this affliction has been found in the use of natural raw foods, and in drinking an ample quantity of carrot and spinach juice.

Lettuce: Lettuce has proved useful in preventing pyorrhoea. The leaves of this vegetable should be chewed everyday immediately after meals for this purpose.

Wheat: Wheat is especially valuable in the prevention and treatment of pyorrhoea. Wheat *chapatis* are usually taken with other foods, and hence, the other food also gets chewed properly. This not only provides the needed exercise for the teeth and gum but also aids in digestion.

Dietary Considerations

The patient should begin the treatment with a short juice fast for three to five days. Oranges and carrots should be used for juices. After the juice fast, the patient should spend the next three to five days on an exclusive fresh fruit diet, taking three meals a day of juicy fruits. Thereafter he may gradually embark upon a balanced diet, with emphasis on fresh fruits, green salads, whole-meal bread, properly cooked vegetables, cheese, nuts, and milk. White bread, white sugar, and all refined and tinned foods must be completely given up. Condiments, sauces, alcohol, coffee, and strong tea, as well as meat and other flesh foods should also be avoided.

Other Measures

During the juice fast, the bowels should be cleansed daily with a warm-water enema. Daily dry friction and a hip bath, as well as breathing and other exercises, should form a part of the morning routine. A hot Epsom salts bath taken twice weekly will also be beneficial.

Rheumatism

*Inflammation and Pain in
Joints, Muscles, Tissues*

The word rheumatism is derived from the Greek word 'rheuma', which means a swelling. It refers to an acute or chronic illness which is characterised by pain and swelling of the muscles, ligaments and tendons, or the joints.

Causes and Symptoms

The onset of the acute variety of rheumatism is characterised by fever, intense soreness, and pain. In the acute muscular type, the area becomes so sensitive that even the weight of bed clothing aggravates the pain. It may settle into a chronic state under a wrong mode of treatment. If the disease is not treated properly in the acute stage, it may become chronic. The symptoms of chronic muscular rheumatism are pain and stiffness of the affected muscles. In the case of chronic articular rheumatism (pain in the joints), pain and stiffness are felt in one or more joints of the body, with swelling in most cases.

The chief cause of rheumatism is the presence of toxic waste products in the blood. The liberal consumption of meat, white bread, sugar, and refined cereals leaves a large residue of toxic wastes in the system. When the vitality is low, the toxic wastes are concentrated around the joints and bony structure, where they form the basis of rheumatism. In certain cases, infection from the teeth, tonsils, and gall-bladder may produce rheumatism. The disease is aggravated by exposure to cold water.

Remedies

Potato Juice: The juice of raw potato is regarded as an excellent remedy for rheumatism. One or two teaspoons of the juice, taken out by pressing mashed raw potatoes, should be taken before meals. This will help to eliminate the toxic condition and relieve rheumatism. The skin of the potato is also an excellent remedy for rheumatism. The skin is exceptionally rich in vital mineral salts, and the water in which the peelings are boiled is one of the best medicines for ailments caused by excess toxic matter in the system. Approximately thirty grams of the potato peelings should be thoroughly washed and boiled in half a litre of water till it is reduced to half. The decoction should then be strained and a glass of the same should be taken three or four times daily.

Bitter Gourd: Bitter gourd is considered beneficial in the treatment of rheumatism. A cup of juice, extracted from the vegetable, should be mixed with a teaspoon of honey, and taken daily for treating this condition. This treatment should be continued for at least three months to provide relief.

Celery: Celery is another effective remedy for rheumatism. A fluid extract of the seeds is more powerful than the raw vegetable. This also has a tonic action on the stomach and kidneys. Five to ten drops of this fluid should be taken in hot water before meals. Powdered seeds can be used as a condiment.

Lemon: Lemons are beneficial in the treatment of rheumatism. The patient should take the juice of two or three lemons each day. This will bring good results.

Walnuts: Walnuts are valuable in rheumatism. They should, however, be thoroughly masticated to achieve beneficial results. Half a dozen can be taken daily in the treatment of this condition.

Rhubarb: The herb rhubarb has been found valuable in rheumatism. The green stalks of this herb should be pounded with an equal quantity of sugar. A teaspoonful should be taken three or four times a day. This remedy seldom fails.

Dietary Considerations

In the case of acute rheumatism, the patient should be put on a short fast of orange juice and water for three or four days. After the juice fast, the patient should be placed on a restricted diet for fourteen days. In this regimen, orange or grapefruit may be taken for breakfast; lunch may consist of raw salad of seasonal vegetables with raisins, prunes, figs, or dates; and dinner may comprise of one or two steamed vegetables. Thereafter, the patient may gradually adopt a well-balanced diet consisting of seeds, nuts, grains, vegetables, and fruits. In case of chronic rheumatism, the patient may be placed on an all-fruit diet for four or five days. He may, thereafter, gradually adopt a well-balanced diet. The patient should take ripe fruits, fresh vegetables, and buttermilk in abundance. He should avoid all meat and fish; white bread, sugar, and refined cereals; rich, indigestible and highly-seasoned foods; tea and coffee; alcohol; sauces, pickles, and condiments.

Other Measures

In the case of acute rheumatism, the bowels should be cleansed daily with a warm-water enema during the first three or four days of the juice fast. Other helpful methods in the treatment of rheumatism are application of heat and hot packs to the affected parts, a hot tub bath, a cabinet steam bath, dry friction, and a sponge bath. Hot Epsom salts baths are also beneficial and should be taken twice a week for three months in case of chronic rheumatism and once weekly thereafter. The affected parts should also be bathed twice daily in hot water containing Epsom salts, after which some olive oil should be applied. Fresh air, deep breathing, and light outdoor exercises are also beneficial. Dampness and cold should be avoided.

Ringworm

A Fungal Disease of the Skin

Ringworm is one of the common skin diseases. The disease is caused by a fungus, a minute form of vegetable plant life that grows on the skin. The disease is more annoying than dangerous.

Causes and Symptoms

Ringworm infection occurs in the scalp, the body, the feet, and the nails. Ringworm of the scalp is common among children

191

because of the lack of protective fatty acids in their scalp. The disease spreads on the skin and extends deeper into the hair roots, and also up along the hair. The affected hair becomes dull and breaks off near its root. This leaves bald spots on the scalp. The patches of ringworm on the body are usually round or oval, with raised pink and scaly rings which show a clean space in the centre. The itching in the infected parts helps to spread infection through the nails to other healthy parts of the body. If it is not treated for a long time, the infection becomes chronic and is then difficult to get rid of.

Ringworm is passed from an infected person to a healthy person by contact. It can also spread by the use of articles such as the towel of an infected person.

Remedies

Papaya: Raw papaya is one of the most effective home remedies for ringworm. The slices of this fruit should be rubbed on the ringworm patches. A paste made from dried papaya seeds can also be applied beneficially on these ringworm patches.

Mustard Seeds: Another effective home remedy for ringworm is mustard seeds. A paste should be prepared from these seeds and applied externally over the ringworm patches after thoroughly washing the skin with sufficient hot water.

Butea Seeds: The seeds of the herb butea are valuable in ringworm. The seeds should be ground to a paste and mixed with a little lime juice. This paste should be applied externally over the skin affected by ringworm.

Cassia Leaves: The leaves of the cassia tree are useful in irritation of the skin and in alleviating swellings and pains. The juice of these leaves or a paste made from them can be applied to ringworm patches with gratifying results.

Holy Basil: The leaves of holy basil are also useful in ringworm. The juice of these leaves should be extracted and applied over ringworm patches.

Turmeric: Turmeric is very effective in the treatment of ringworm. The juice of raw turmeric should be applied externally to the parts of the skin affected by ringworm. Simultaneously, one teaspoon of turmeric juice mixed with an equal quantity of honey should be taken orally.

Raw Vegetable Juices: Raw vegetable juices, especially carrot juice in combination with spinach juice, have proved beneficial in the treatment of ringworm. The formula proportions considered helpful in this combination are 300 ml of carrot juice and 200 ml of spinach juice to make 500 ml or half a litre of juice.

Dietary Considerations

To begin with, the patient should adopt an all-fruit diet for about five days. He should take three meals a day of fresh juicy fruits such as apples, oranges, papayas, pineapples, and pomegranates at five-hourly intervals. This will help eliminate morbid matter from the body and lead to substantial improvement.

Fruits and salt-free raw or steamed vegetables with whole-wheat *chapatis* may be taken after the all-fruit diet. After a few days curd and milk may be added to the diet. The patient may, there-after, gradually embark upon a well-balanced diet with emphasis on seeds, nuts, wholegrain cereals, raw or lightly cooked vegetables, and fresh fruits.

The patient should avoid tea, coffee, all condiments and highly flavoured dishes, as well as sugar, white flour products, and tinned or bottled foods.

Other Measures

A warm-water enema may be administered to cleanse the bowels during the all-fruit diet. The patient should get as much fresh air as possible. He should drink plenty of water and bathe twice daily. The skin, with the exception of the part affected with ringworm, should be vigorously rubbed with the palms of the hands before taking a bath.

Coconut oil may be applied to the parts with ringworm spots. It will help the skin to stay soft. Sunbathing is also beneficial and should be resorted to early in the morning, at the first light of dawn. A light mudpack applied over the areas of the ringworm is also helpful. The pack should be applied for half an hour, twice daily.

Scurvy

Vitamin C Deficiency Disease

Scurvy is, perhaps, the oldest known deficiency disease. However, its specific relationship to ascorbic acid was not recognised until the 20th century. The disease is common among children and is often mistaken for rheumatism, rickets, or paralysis.

Scurvy was widely prevalent in the 19th century among sailors on long voyages. They often subsisted for long periods on salt, fish, meats, and breadstuffs, and were entirely deprived of any fresh food. Later, limes and lemons were included in the supplies, since they were found to be anti-scorbutic, that is, they prevented scurvy.

Causes and Symptoms

The onset of scurvy is gradual. The first signs of the disease are exhaustion and general weakness. At the later stages, there is bleeding of the gums, because the lack of vitamin C (ascorbic acid) makes the capillaries fragile and their rupture is common. This may lead to extensive haemorrhaging.

Scurvy is caused by lack of vitamin C or ascorbic acid. Inadequate intake of fresh fruits and vegetables can lead to this condition. Another important cause of scurvy is stress which increases the utilisation of ascorbic acid.

Remedies

Indian Gooseberry: The Indian gooseberry is one of the most effective home remedies for scurvy. It is the richest source of vitamin C. Dry *amla* should be powdered with an equal quantity of sugar. This powder should be given in doses of one teaspoon, three times daily, with milk.

Lime and Lemon: The use of lime and lemon is highly beneficial in the prevention and treatment of scurvy. Being rich sources of vitamin C, lime and lemon are regarded as foods of exceptional therapeutic value. They have saved the lives of innumerable crews of ocean-going vessels from scurvy. The juice of one lime or lemon mixed in a glass of water, with a teaspoon of honey, should be taken for treating this condition.

Mango Powder: Another effective remedy for scurvy is the use of *aamchur*, a popular article of diet in Indian houses, consisting of green mangoes — skinned, stoned, cut into pieces, dried in the sun and powdered. Fifteen grams of *aamchur* are believed to be equivalent to thirty grams of good lime on account of its citric content.

Potato: Potato is regarded as an excellent food remedy for scurvy. It contains up to 17 mg of vitamin C, can be found in 100 mg of potatoes. It has been noted that scurvy in Europe has become more and more uncommon with the progress of potato cultivation and it makes its appearance only when the crop fails.

Jaundice Berry: Jaundice berry is a valuable herbal remedy for scurvy. The leaves of the plant are anti-scorbutic or anti-scurvy. A decoction of the leaves can be prepared by boiling 15 gm of dried leaves in 500 ml of water till it is reduced by one-third. About 150 to 175 ml of the decoction can be taken at a time. The juice of the berry is also beneficial and can be taken in doses of 2 to 4 ml.

Dietary Considerations

The most important factor in the prevention and treatment of scurvy is proper feeding. After birth, all children should be breast-fed wherever possible. Mother's milk is pure and fresh and contains, in correct proportions, most of the nutrients necessary for the growth and development of the baby. If, for any reason, it is not possible to breast-feed the baby, he or she should be fed either on cow's milk or commercially available milk formulas. After the age of one year, the child may be given fruits and vegetable juices, besides milk and occasional intake of wholemeal bread. After the age of two years, the child can be gradually allowed to embark upon a well-balanced diet, with emphasis on fruits, steamed vegetables, wholegrain cereals, and milk.

Diet also plays an important role in the prevention and treatment of scurvy in adults. The patient should take a well-balanced diet consisting of seeds, nuts, grains, vegetables, and fruits. This diet should be supplemented with certain special foods such as milk, vegetable oils, and honey. The patient should be given liberal quantities of foods rich in vitamin C. This vitamin is found in fresh fruits and vegetables. The daily requirement of this vitamin is between 10–20 mg daily. It can be taken in tablet form, if necessary.

Other Measures

The patient should also undertake outdoor exercises like walking, swimming, and cycling. He should sleep in a well-ventilated room, and spend as much time as possible in the fresh air.

Sexual Impotence

Sex is a basic instinct like hunger. Sexual activity, however, demands complete concentration and relaxation. It cannot be performed in haste and tension. Persons who are usually tense and overoccupied are unable to follow these norms. Many persons, therefore, suffer from sexual dysfunctions. The most common male sexual dysfunction is impotence.

Causes and Symptoms

Impotence takes three forms. There is primary impotence when the man's erectile dysfunction is there from the very beginning of sexual activity and he simply cannot have an erection. Secondary impotence is the commonest and this implies that the man can normally attain an erection but fails on one or more occasions in between normal activity. The third form is associated with advancing age.

Sexual impotence may result from psychological illness such as depression which lowers both sexual drive and erectile function, tiredness, alcohol abuse, the therapeutic use of oestrogens, paralysis of parasympathetic nerves by drugs or permanent damage to them, and diabetes. Other causes of impotence include a devitalised condition of the system in general. The main problem of secondary impotence is the apprehension created by an earlier failure, which generates a good deal of anxiety for the next time.

Remedies

Garlic: Garlic is one of the most remarkable home remedies found beneficial in the treatment of sexual impotence. It is a natural and harmless aphrodisiac. According to an eminent sexologist of the United States, garlic has a pronounced aphrodisiac effect. It is a tonic for loss of sexual power due to any cause, and for sexual debility and impotency resulting from sexual overindulgence and nervous exhaustion. Two to three cloves of raw garlic should be chewed daily.

Onion: Onion is another important aphrodisiac food, second only to garlic. It increases libido and strengthens the reproductory organs. The white variety of onion is, however, more useful for this purpose.

Carrot: Carrots are considered valuable in impotence. For better results, about 150 gm of carrots, chopped finely, should be taken with a half-boiled egg, dipped in a tablespoon of honey, once daily for a month or two. This recipe increases sexual stamina.

Lady's Fingers: Lady's fingers are another tonic for improving sexual vigour. It has been mentioned in ancient Indian literature that persons who take five to ten grams of the root powder of this vegetable with a glass of milk and two teaspoons of ground *mishri* daily, will never lose sexual vigour.

Asparagus: The dried roots of asparagus are used in Unani medicine as an aphrodisiac. They are available in the market as *safed musli*. Fifteen grams of roots boiled in one cup of milk should be taken twice daily. The regular use of this remedy is valuable in impotency and premature ejaculation.

Drumstick: A soup made with about fifteen grams of drumstick flowers boiled in 250 ml milk is very useful as a sexual tonic in the treatment of sexual debility. It is also useful in functional sterility in both males and females. The powder of the dry bark is also valuable in impotency, premature ejaculation, and thinness of semen. About 120 gm of the powder of the dry bark should be boiled in half a litre of water for about half an hour. Thirty grams of this powder, mixed with a tablespoon of honey, should be taken three times daily for a month.

Ginger: The juice extracted from ginger is a valuable aphrodisiac and beneficial in the treatment of sexual weakness. For better results, half a teaspoon of ginger juice should be taken with a half-boiled egg and honey, once daily at night, for a month. It is said to relieve impotency, premature ejaculation, and spermatorrhoea.

Dried Dates: Dried dates are a highly-strengthening food. Pounded and mixed with almonds, pistachio nuts, and quince seeds in equal quantities, about 100 gm should be taken daily as an effective medicine for increasing sexual power.

Raisins: Black raisins are useful for restoration of sexual vigour. They should be boiled with milk after being washed thoroughly in tepid water. This will make them swollen and sweet. Eating of these raisins should be followed by the intake of milk. Starting with 30 gm of raisins, followed by 200 ml of milk three times daily, the quantity of raisins should be gradually increased to 50 gm each time.

Dietary Considerations

Diet is an important factor in treating sexual impotence. To begin with, the patient should adopt an exclusive fresh-fruit diet for five to seven days, taking three meals a day of fresh juicy fruits at five-hourly intervals. After the all-fruit diet, he may gradually embark upon a well-balanced diet consisting of seeds, nuts, grains, vegetables, and fruits, with generous use of special rejuvenative foods such as whey, sour milk — particularly goat's mailk, millet, garlic, honey, cold-pressed vegetable oils, and brewer's yeast. The patient should avoid smoking, alcohol, tea, and coffee; and all processed, canned, refined, and denatured foods, especially white sugar and white flour, and products made from them.

Other Measures

A vigorous massage all over the body is highly beneficial in the treatment of impotence, as it helps to revive muscular vigour which is essential for nervous energy. The nerves of the genital organs are controlled by the pelvic region. Hence a cold hip bath for ten minutes in the morning or evening is very effective. Every effort should be made to build up the general health level to the highest degree, and fresh air and outdoor exercises are essential for the success of the treatment. *Yogasanas* such as *dhanurasana, sarvangasana,* and *halasana* are also highly beneficial.

Sinusitis

Inflammation of the Sinuses

Sinusitis refers to an inflammation of the mucous membrane lining the paranasal sinuses. It often follows à common cold, influenza, and other general infections. Infecting germs sometimes find their way into these sinuses or chambers on either side of the nasal passage, leading to sinus trouble.

Causes and Symptoms

The symptoms of sinusitis are excessive or constant sneezing; a running nose; blockage of one or both nostrils; headaches and pressure around the head, eyes, and face. Sinus headaches are usually felt in the forehead and in the face just below the eyes.

The patient may suffer from low grade fever, lack of appetite, and difficulty in breathing.

Sinusitis results from the inflammation of the sinus passages and oversecretion of mucus by the membranes lining the nose and throat.

Remedies

Mango: The liberal use of mangoes during the season is considered an effective remedy for prevention and treatment of sinusitis. Mangoes contribute towards formation of healthy epithelium, thereby preventing frequent attacks of common infections like sinusitis. This is attributable to a high concentration of vitamin A in the fruit.

Garlic and Onion: The use of pungent foods like garlic and onion is one of the most effective remedies for sinus problems. One should begin with small mild doses and increase them gradually. Beneficial results can also be achieved by adding these herbs in moderate amounts to regular meals.

Fenugreek: The seeds of fenugreek are another effective remedy for sinusitis. A tea prepared by boiling one teaspoon of seeds in 250 ml of water till it is reduced to half, will help the body to produce perspiration, dispel toxicity, and shorten the period of fever in the acute stage of the disease. Upto four cups should be taken daily. The quantity should be reduced as the condition improves.

Cumin Seeds: A teaspoon of black cumin seeds tied in a thin cotton cloth can provide relief when inhaled. The condition can also be relieved by taking a mixture of 100 gm of roasted and ground cumin seeds and 200 gm of pure honey.

Vegetable Juices: Carrot juice, taken separately or in combination with juices of beet and cucumber, or with spinach juice, has been found beneficial in the treatment of sinus trouble. In the case of combined juices, 100 ml each of beet and cucumber juices, or 200 ml of spinach juice, should be mixed with 300 ml of carrot juice to make 500 ml or half a litre of the mixed juice.

Vitamins A and C: A diet rich in vitamin A is the best insurance against cold and sinus trouble. Vitamin A is the 'membrane conditioner' and it helps build healthy mucous membranes in the nose and throat. Some of the valuable sources of this vitamin are whole milk, curds, egg yolk, pumpkin, carrots, leafy vegetables, tomatoes, mangoes, and papaya. When the sinus trouble has already developed, relief can be obtained by taking vitamin A in large therapeutic doses of 25,000 IU per day. Vitamin C has also proved beneficial in the treatment of sinusitis and the patient should take one gram of this vitamin per day in two therapeutic doses of 500 mg each.

Dietary Considerations

In the acute stage of the disease, when fever is present, the patient should abstain from all solid foods and drink only fresh fruit and vegetable juices diluted with warm water on a 50:50 basis. After the fever subsides, he may adopt a low-calorie, raw fruit and vegetable diet with plenty of raw juices. Once the acute symptoms are over, the patient may gradually embark upon a well-balanced diet, with emphasis on seeds, nuts, grains, vegetables, and fruits. In persistent chronic conditions, repeated short juice fasts may be undertaken for a week or so at intervals of two months. The patient should avoid fried and starchy foods, white sugar, white flour, rice, macaroni products, pies, cakes, and candies.

Other Measures

A cold application over the sinus will give great relief, while alternate hot and cold applications also prove beneficial. Take pans of hot and cold water, bathe the whole face with hot water—as hot as you can bear—and then apply cold water for a short duration. Nasal inhalation of steam for five minutes every hour will also give relief. Plenty of sleep, adequate rest, and fresh air are essential in the treatment of sinus trouble. Patients should avoid the use of perfumes and strongly scented hair oil.

Sore Throat

Inflammation of the Throat

Sore throat refers to the inflammation of the pharynx or back of the throat. It occurs frequently when a person has a cold or an attack of influenza. This inflammation may also involve the tonsils and adenoids.

Causes and Symptoms

In the case of an acute sore throat, the patient complains of pain, irritation, and inflammation in the throat; followed by chills, fever, and some hoarseness or laryngitis. The lymph glands along the sides of the neck may become swollen and tender. The back of the throat may become very red and even covered with a greyish-white membrane. The patient may find difficulty in swallowing, especially during the acute stage. There may also be some postnatal discharge if the inflammation has spread to the nasal passages.

The main causes of a sore throat are common cold and influenza. Other causes include sinusitis, measles, diphtheria, and even leukaemia in rare cases.

Remedies

Mango Bark: Mango bark is efficacious in the treatment of a sore throat and other throat disorders. Its fluid, which is extracted by grinding, can be applied locally with beneficial results. It can also be used as a throat gargle. This gargle is prepared by mixing 10 ml of the fluid extract with 125 ml of water.

Belleric Myroblan: The herb belleric myroblan is valuable in sore throat. A mixture of two grams of the pulp of the fruit, a quarter teaspoon of salt, half a teaspoon of powdered long pepper, and two teaspoons of honey should be administered in the treatment of this condition. The fried fruit can also be roasted after covering it with wheat flour, and used as a cure for a sore throat.

Bishop's Weed: Bishop's weed is valuable in treating a sore throat. An infusion of the seeds mixed with common salt can be used beneficially as a gargle in an acute condition caused by a cold.

Cinnamon: Cinnamon is regarded as an effective remedy for a sore throat resulting from a cold. One teaspoon of coarsely powdered cinnamon, boiled in a glass of water with a pinch of pepper powder, and two teaspoons of honey can be taken as a medicine in the treatment of this condition. Two or three drops of cinnamon oil, mixed with a teaspoon of honey, also give immense relief.

Fenugreek Seeds: A gargle prepared from fenugreek seeds has been found to be a very effective remedy for treating a sore throat. To prepare this gargle, two tablespoons of fenugreek seeds should be put in a litre of cold water and allowed to simmer for half an hour over a low flame. This should then be allowed to cool to a bearable temperature, strained, and then used entirely as a gargle.

Henna: The leaves of henna are useful in a sore throat. A decoction of the leaves can be used as a gargle for this purpose.

Holy Basil: The leaves of holy basil have also been found beneficial in the treatment of this condition. Water boiled with basil leaves should be taken as a drink, and also used as a gargle to relieve a sore throat.

Kantakari: The herb *kantakari* has proved valuable in sore throat. An extract of the plant should be used as a gargle for this purpose. This extract is prepared by continuously boiling the plant in about two litres of water after washing it thoroughly.

Liquorice: Liquorice is a recognized home remedy for sore throat in all parts of India. A small piece of raw liquorice should be chewed or sucked for treating this condition. The healing property of the herb soothes inflammation quickly.

Sage: Sage is another effective remedy for a sore throat. Half a litre of boiling water should be poured on a handful of sage leaves. When moderately cool, a little vinegar and honey should be added according to taste. This mixture should be used as a gargle. A teaspoon of this mixture can also be taken internally at the same time.

Tea Decoction: A decoction made from tea leaves is very beneficial in the treatment of a sore throat. This decoction, mixed with a pinch of salt, should be used as a gargle. It can be used two or three times daily for obtaining relief. It is not necessary to use fresh leaves for this purpose. Boiling water can be poured over used tea leaves in the tea jug and this decoction used as a gargle.

Tamarind: Tamarind is also beneficial in the treatment of this condition. Tamarind water should be used as a gargle. A powder of the dry leaves and an infusion of the bark can also be used for preparation of a gargle for treating sore throat.

Dietary Considerations

A person suffering from a sore throat should fast on orange juice and water for three to five days, depending on the severity of the condition.

When the severe symptoms subside, the patient may adopt an all-fruit diet for three or four further days. Thereafter, he may adopt a well-balanced diet, with emphasis on seeds, nuts, grains, raw vegetables, and fresh fruits.

Other Measures

During the initial juice and water fast, the bowels should be cleansed daily with a warm-water enema. This should be done twice daily in more serious cases. A wet pack should be applied to the throat at two-hourly intervals during the day, and one at night. The procedure is to wring out some linen cloth in cold water, wrap it two or three times around the affected part, and cover it with flannel. Gargles may be done several times. A hot Epsom salts bath, taken daily during this period, will be highly beneficial. Dry friction, deep breathing, and other exercises should form part of the daily health regimen.

Stress

Mental Tension

The term stress implies any condition that harms the body or the mind. The most common disorders associated with stress are heart disease, diabetes, headache, and peptic ulcer.

Causes and Symptoms

The body and the mind react to any stress factor. A large number of physical changes take place when a person is under stress. The brain and nervous system become intensely active; the pupils of the eye dilate; digestion slows down; muscles become tense; the heart starts pumping blood harder and faster; blood pressure increases; breathing becomes faster; hormones such as adrenaline are released into the system along with glucose from the liver; and sweating starts. All these changes take place in a split second under the direction of the nervous system. If the stress factors are removed immediately, no harm accrues and all the changes are reversed. Stress in its earlier and reversible stage leads to poor sleep, bad temper, continual grumbling, domestic conflict, repeated minor sickness, accident proneness, a feeling of frustration, and increase in alcoholic intake.

Stress may be caused by a variety of factors both outside the body and within. External factors include loud noises, blinding lights, extreme heat or cold, X-rays and other forms of radiation, drugs, chemicals, bacterial and various toxic substances, pain, and inadequate nutrition. The factors from within the body include hate, envy, fear, or jealousy.

Remedies

Holy Basil: The leaves of holy basil have been found beneficial in the treatment of stress. They are regarded as an anti-stress agent. Recent studies have shown that the leaves protect against stress significantly. It has been suggested that even healthy persons should chew twelve leaves of basil twice a day, morning and evening, for preventing stress.

Sage: The herb sage is considered valuable in stress. A tea prepared from the leaves of this plant should be given in the treatment of this condition. This tea is prepared by pouring a cup of boiling water over one teaspoon of dried sage leaves. The water should be covered and infused for several minutes. It should then be strained and sweetened with honey, if desired. In the case of fresh leaves, a tablespoon of coarsely chopped sage leaves should be used and tea prepared in the same way.

Nutrients: Certain nutrients have proved beneficial in relieving stress. These are vitamins A and B; and minerals such as calcium, potassium, and magnesium which reduce the feeling of irritability and anxiety. Vitamin A is found in green and yellow vegetables. Some of the valuable sources of vitamin B are cashew nuts, green leafy vegetables, yeast, sprouts, and bananas. An element of vitamin B complex, pantothenic acid, is especially important in preventing stress. It has a deep effect on the adrenal glands and the immune system; an adequate amount of this vitamin, along with vitamin A, can help prevent many of the changes caused by stress.

Potassium deficiencies are associated with breathlessness, fatigue, insomnia, and low blood sugar. Potassium is essential for healthy heart muscles. Nuts and whole grains are good sources of this mineral. Calcium is a natural sedative. Deficiencies can cause fatigue, nervousness, and tension. Dairy products, eggs, almonds, and soya beans are rich sources of this mineral. Magnesium is known as nature's tranquilliser and is associated with the prevention of heart attacks. It is found in many fruits, vegetables, seeds, dates, and prunes.

Other Foods: There are many foods which help in meeting the demands of stress and should be taken regularly by the patients.

These include yoghurt, blackstrap molasses, seeds, and sprouts. Yoghurt is rich in vitamins A, D, and the B complex group. It relieves migraine, insomnia, and cramps associated with menstruation. Blackstrap molasses, a by-product of the sugar-refining process, is rich in iron and B vitamins. It guards against anaemia and is good for heart disease. Seeds such as alfalfa, sunflower, pumpkins, and sprouts are rich in calcium and quite effective as deterrents of listlessness and anxiety.

Dietary Considerations

In dealing with stress, the lifestyle of the patient needs a complete overhaul. He should be placed on an optimum diet, and be encouraged to take regular exercise and adequate rest. If this is done, many diseases caused by stress can be eliminated. Diet plays an important role in the prevention and healing of stress-induced diseases. Certain foods associated with stress and anxiety should be scrupulously avoided. These foods are caffeine in coffee and many soft drinks, salt, sugar, cigarettes, and alcohol.

Other Measures

Regular physical exercise plays an important role in the fight against stress. It not only keeps the body physically and mentally fit, but also provides recreation and mental relaxation. Recreation and rest are also important. The patient should set a definite time for recreational activities, and should take a holiday at regular intervals. Above all, he should simplify his style of living to eliminate unnecessary stress.

Tonsillitis

Inflammation of the Tonsils

Tonsillitis refers to acute inflammation of the tonsils, which lie, one on each side of the throat. Chronic tonsillitis is a term applied to cases in which there is enlargement of the tonsils accompanied by repeated attacks of infection.

Causes and Symptoms

The main symptoms of tonsillitis are sore throat, fever, headache, pain in various parts of the body, difficulty in swallowing, and general weakness. The tonsils are seen to be inflamed and red when the mouth is opened wide. In many cases, spots of pus exude from them. Externally, the tonsillar lymph glands which lie just behind the angle of the jaw are tender and enlarged. In severe cases, there may be pain in the ear.

The chief cause of tonsillitis is a toxic condition of the system which is brought to a head by a sudden lowering of vitality, resulting from exposure and sudden chill. The tonsils enlarge and get inflamed when the toxins cannot be got rid of through the normal channels of elimination such as the bowels, kidneys, and skin. A throat affliction of this kind is also associated with and is the result of chronic constipation, when toxins are reabsorbed into the bloodstream.

Remedies

Lime: Lime is one of the most effective remedies in the treatment of acute tonsillitis. A fresh lime squeezed in a glass of warm water, with four teaspoons of honey and a quarter teaspoon of common salt, should be sipped slowly in such cases.

Milk: Milk has been found valuable in tonsillitis. A glass of pure boiled milk, mixed with a pinch of turmeric powder and pepper powder, should be taken every night for three nights in the treatment of this condition. It will bring beneficial results.

Vegetable Juices: Juices of carrot, beet, and cucumber, taken individually or in combination, are especially beneficial. The formula proportion recommended, when used in combination is 300 ml of carrot juice, 100 ml of beet juice, and 100 ml of cucumber juice.

Banafsha Flowers: Banafsha flowers, botanically known as *Viola odorata,* are beneficial in the treatment of tonsillitis. About 12 gm of these flowers should be boiled in 50 ml of milk. This milk should be taken hot after being filtered. The filtered banafsha can also be lightly fried in *ghee* and worn round the throat as a poultice at night.

Fenugreek Seeds: A gargle made from fenugreek seeds is very effective in severe cases of tonsillitis. To make such a gargle, two tablespoons of fenugreek seeds should be allowed to simmer for half an hour in a litre of water and then set aside to cool. The entire quantity should be used the same day as a soothing gargle. It will have beneficial results.

Dietary Considerations

To begin with, the patient should fast for three to five days, by which time the serious symptoms should subside. Nothing but water and orange juice should be taken during this time.

After the acute symptoms of tonsillitis are over, the patient should adopt an all-fruit diet for the next three or four days. Thereafter he may gradually embark upon a well-balanced diet, with emphasis on seeds, nuts, grains, vegetables, and fruits. The patient should avoid spices and condiments as they tend to irritate the throat. Sour substances like curds, buttermilk, and fried foods should also be avoided.

Other Measures

Daily dry friction and a hip bath, as well as breathing and other exercises, should all form part of the daily health regimen. The bowels should be cleansed daily with a warm-water enema during the period of fasting. A cold pack should be applied to the throat at two-hourly intervals during the day. A hot Epsom salts bath taken everyday or every other day will also be beneficial.

Toothache

Pain in a Tooth

The teeth are an amazing balance of form and function, aesthetic beauty and engineering. Good teeth are an important part of one's health and appearance. Toothache is a common problem.

Causes and Symptoms

A toothache may be sharp, throbbing, shooting, or constant. If the tooth is not properly treated, it will eventually have to be extracted.

The main cause of toothache is tooth decay which results from a faulty diet. Perhaps the greatest curse and cause of tooth decay is the consumption of candy, soft drinks, pastries, refined carbohydrates, and sugar in all forms. Bacteria in the mouth break sugar down into acids, which combine with the calcium in the enamel to cause decay or erosion.

Remedies

Garlic: Garlic is one of most effective of several home remedies for toothache. A clove of garlic with a little rock salt should be placed on the affected tooth. It will relieve the pain and, sometimes, may even cure it. A clove should also be chewed daily in the morning. It will make the teeth strong and healthy.

Onion: Latest research has confirmed the bactericidal properties of onion. If a person consumes one raw onion every day by thorough mastication, he will be protected from a host of tooth disorders. Chewing raw onion for three minutes is sufficient to kill all the germs in the mouth. Toothache is often allayed by placing a small piece of onion on the bad tooth or gum.

Lime: Lime, as a rich source of vitamin C, is useful in maintaining the health of the teeth and other bones of the body. It prevents decay and loosening of the teeth, dental caries, toothache, and bleeding of the gums.

Wheat Grass: The juice of wheat grass acts as an excellent mouthwash for tooth decay and toothache. Wheat grass can be chewed with beneficial results. It draws out toxins from the gums and thus checks bacterial growth.

Asafoetida: The use of asafoetida has been found useful in alleviating toothache. It should be pestled in lemon juice and slightly heated. A cotton swab should be soaked in this lotion and placed in the cavity of the tooth. It will relieve pain quickly.

Bay Berry: A paste of the bark of bay berry should be made with vinegar. This paste, applied on the affected tooth, will relieve the toothache. It can also be applied beneficially on the gums for strengthening them.

Clove: The use of a clove in toothache reduces pain. It also helps to decrease infection due to its antiseptic properties. Clove oil, applied to a cavity in a decayed tooth, also relieves toothache.

Pepper: A mixture of a pinch of pepper powder and a quarter teaspoon of common salt is an excellent dentrifice. Its daily use prevents dental caries, foul breath, bleeding from the gums, painful gums, and toothaches. It cures the increased sensitiveness of the teeth. A pinch of pepper powder mixed with clove oil can be put on the caries to alleviate the toothache.

Dietary Considerations

Diet plays a vital role in dental health. The condition of the teeth after they are formed depends upon the foods one eats from day to day. Dental decay, the destruction of the bone around the teeth, and infection of the gums can be prevented with an appropriate diet. In fact, with a proper diet, the teeth and jaw bones can be made harder and healthier as the years go by.

It is important to restrict one's sugar intake, and to ensure that the diet includes plenty of raw vegetables and wholewheat bread. Whole foods are ideal for the teeth. Fibreless refined foods allow particles to accumulate on the teeth in a sticky mass where they can do great harm. The gums need friction to keep them firm and whole foods also help remove plaque. They are therefore called 'detergent foods' by some dentists.

In preventing tooth decay, what one eats is no doubt important but equally important is when one eats. Frequent small snacks are very harmful to teeth, as they produce an acid medium in which the bacteria thrive. The number of times one eats sugar is one of the most important factors in determining the rate of decay. For this reason, it is better to eat sweets at the end of a meal rather than between meals.

Other Measures

Proper cleaning of the teeth is very essential to prevent tooth decay and consequent toothache. There are many theories on how best to clean the teeth. The consensus of dental opinion, however, seems to back using a circular motion with the brush, so as to ensure that all dental surfaces are cleaned. One should not be afraid to touch the gums with the brush, as this gentle stimulation improves the blood circulation in the gums.

Tuberculosis

Koch's Disease

Tuberculosis is a serious disease. It is caused by a tiny germ called tubercle bacillus. The germ enters into the body through the nose, mouth, and the windpipe, and settles down in the lungs. It multiplies by millions and produces small raised spots called tubercles.

Causes and Symptoms

Tuberculosis may occur anywhere in the body but, more commonly, it affects the lungs, intestines, bones, and glands. Pulmonary tuberculosis or tuberculosis of the lungs is by far the most common type of tuberculosis. It tends to consume the body and the patient loses strength, colour, and weight. Other symptoms are a rise in temperature—especially in the evening, a persistent cough and hoarseness, difficulty in breathing, pain in the shoulders, indigestion, chest pain, and blood in the sputum.

Lowered resistance or devitalisation of the system is the chief cause of this disease. Lowered resistance can result from intake of improper and inadequate foods, and living in ill-ventilated houses. Other causes include exposure to cold, loss of sleep, impure air, a sedentary life, overwork, use of tobacco, liquor and other harmful drinks. These factors prepare the ground for the growth of germs of various kinds, including tubercle bacillus. These germs may be present in the body but are quite harmless for those who are endowed with vitality and natural resistance.

Remedies

Milk Diet: The chief therapeutic agent needed for the treatment of tuberculosis is calcium. Milk is the richest food source for the supply of organic calcium to the body and should be taken liberally. In fact, an exclusive milk diet is considered highly valuable in tuberculosis. However, a preparatory fast for three days, consisting of raw juices, preferably, orange juice, is essential before the milk diet is begun. The procedure is to take half a glass of orange juice diluted with an equal quantity of water every two hours from 8 a.m. to 8 p.m. For the full milk diet, the patient should have a glass of milk every two hours from 8 a.m. to 8 p.m. on the first day, followed by a glass and a half every hour on the second day. Thereafter, the quantity can be gradually increased until the patient takes a glass every half an hour. Usually, six litres of milk should be taken every day. In the case of women, five litres should be sufficient.

Raw milk, that is, milk which has not been pasteurised, produces the best results, provided it is clean and pure. Milk should be kept cool and away from dust, flies, odours, and sunlight. It should be gently stirred before use to ensure an even distribution of cream. It should be sipped very slowly so as to be thoroughly mixed with saliva which dilutes it and, to a great extent, promotes its digestion.

Nearly eight to six weeks of a full milk diet is necessary for the success of the treatment. A considerable amount of rest is necessary with a milk diet and the patient should lie down for about two hours twice a day.

Custard Apple: Custard apple is regarded as one of the most valuable remedies for tuberculosis. It is said to contain the qualities of rejuvenating drugs. Ayurvedic practitioners prepare a fermented liquor called *sitaphalasava* from this fruit, when in season, for use as a medicine in the treatment of this disease. The pulp of two custard apples and twenty-five seedless raisins should be boiled in water on a slow fire. When about one-third of the water is left, it should be filtered, and then mixed with two teaspoons of powdered sugar candy, and a quarter teaspoon each of the powder of cardamom, cinnamon, and certain other condiments.

Indian Gooseberry: The Indian gooseberry is another valuable remedy for tuberculosis. A tablespoon each of fresh *amla* juice and honey, mixed together, should be taken every morning in treating this disease. Its regular use will promote vigour and vitality in the body within a few days.

Pineapple: Pineapple juice is beneficial in the treatment of tuberculosis. It has been found to be effective in dissolving mucus and aiding recovery. This juice was used regularly in the past in treating this disease when it was more common than it is at present. One glass of pineapple juice is recommended daily.

Banana: Bananas are considered useful in tuberculosis. According to Dr J. Montelvz of Brazil, South America, the juice of the plantain or the ordinary cooking bananas works miracles in the cure of tuberculosis. He claims to have cured patients in an advanced stage of this disease with frequent cough, abundant expectoration and high fever in two months, by this treatment.

Orange: Oranges are useful in the treatment of tuberculosis. A glass of orange juice should be mixed with a pinch of salt and a tablespoon of honey and taken daily by the patient. Due to its saline action in the lungs, it eases expectoration and protects the body from secondary infections.

Drumstick: A soup prepared from drumstick leaves has been found valuable in this disease. This soup is prepared by adding a handful of leaves to 200 ml of water which has been heated to a boiling point. The water should then be allowed to boil for five minutes more. After that it should be removed from the fire and allowed to cool. A little salt, pepper, and lime juice may be added to this soup. This drink should be taken first thing every morning.

Bottle Gourd: The use of bottle gourd is considered an effective remedy for tuberculosis. According to Dr C.D. Mehta of Bengal T.B. Sanitorium, bottle gourd is one of the best vegetables for tuberculosis patients. He has carried out extensive research which confirms that regular use of cooked bottle gourd helps in developing immunity against tubercular germs.

Mint: The fresh juice of mint has also been found useful in this disease. A teaspoon of this juice, mixed with two teaspoons of pure malt vinegar and an equal quantity of honey, should be stirred in 120 ml of carrot juice. This should be given as a medicinal tonic thrice daily in the treatment of tuberculosis. It liquefies the sputum, nourishes the lungs, increases body resistance against infection, and prevents the harmful effects of anti-tubercular drugs.

Dietary Considerations

The patient should avoid all devitalising foods such as white bread, white sugar, and refined cereals; puddings and pies; and tinned, canned, and preserved foods. He should also avoid strong tea, coffee, condiments, pickles, and sauces.

Other Measures

The patient should completely rest his mind and body. Any type of stress will delay healing. Fresh air is always important in curing the disease, and the patient should spend most of the time in the open air and sleep in a well-ventilated room. Sunshine is also essential as tubercle bacilli are killed rapidly by exposure to the sun's rays. Other beneficial steps towards curing the disease are avoidance of strain, slow massage, deep breathing, and a light occupation to ensure mental diversion.

Underweight

Being thin or underweight, like being overweight, is a relative term, being based on the ideal weight for a given height, built, and sex. A person can be regarded as moderately underweight if he or she weighs ten per cent below the ideal body weight and markedly so if the weight is twenty per cent below the ideal.

Causes and Symptoms

Thinness due to an inadequate caloric intake is a serious condition, especially in young people. They often feel easily fatigued, have poor physical stamina and low resistance to infection. Diseases like tuberculosis, respiratory disorders, pneumonia, circulatory diseases like heart disorders, cerebral haemorrhage, nephritis, typhoid fever, and cancer are quite common among them.

Thinness may be due to inadequate nutrition or excessive bodily activity, or both. Emotional factors or bad eating habits such as skipping meals, small meals, habitual fasting, and inadequate exercise can also cause it. Other factors include inadequate digestion and absorption of food due to a wrong dietary pattern for a particular metabolism, metabolic disturbances such as an overactive thyroid, and hereditary tendencies. Disorders such as chronic dyspepsia, chronic diarrhoea, presence of intestinal worms, liver disorders, diabetes mellitus, insomnia, constipation, and sexual disorders can also lead to thinness.

Remedies

Musk Melon: Musk melon is one of the most effective home remedies for thinness. If the melon cure is properly carried out, a rapid gain in weight can usually be achieved. In this mode of treatment, only musk melons are taken three times during the day for forty days or more. In the beginning, only three kilograms of melons are taken daily for three days. Then the quantity is increased by one kilogram daily till it is sufficient to appease the hunger. Only the sweet and fresh fruits of the best variety are used in the treatment.

Mango-Milk Cure: The mango-milk cure is also an ideal treatment for thinness. For this mode of treatment, ripe and sweet mangoes should always be selected. They should be taken thrice a day—morning, afternoon, and evening. Two medium sized mangoes should be taken first and then followed by a glass of milk. Mango is rich in sugar but deficient in protein. On the other hand, milk is rich in protein but deficient in sugar. The deficiency of one is made up by the other. Mango thus combines very well with milk and an exclusive mango-milk diet taken for at least one month, will lead to improvement in health and vigour and gain in weight.

Milk Cure: An exclusive milk diet for rapid gain of weight has been advocated by some nature cure practitioners. At the beginning of this mode of treatment, the patient should fast for three days on warm water and lime juice so as to cleanse the system. Thereafter, he should have a glass of milk every two hours from 8 a.m. to 8 p.m. on the first day, a glass every hour and half the next day, and a glass every hour the third day. Then the quantity of milk should be gradually increased so as to take a glass every half an hour from 8 a.m. to 8 p.m., if such a quantity can be tolerated fairly comfortably.

Figs: Figs are an excellent remedy for increasing weight in case of thinness. The high percentage of the rapidly assimilable sugar in this fruit make it a strengthening and fattening food. Three dried figs soaked in water should be taken twice daily.

Raisins: Raisins are a good food for those who wish to gain weight. Thirty grams a day may be taken for this purpose.

Nutrients: Nutrients which help to keep the nerves relaxed are of utmost importance as nervousness causes all the muscles to become tense, and the energy which goes into the tensing wastefully uses up a great deal of food. Although all vitamins and minerals are required for relaxation, the most important once are vitamin D and B_6, calcium, and magnesium. The richest sources of vitamin D are milk, cod-liver oil, and rays of the sun. Calcium is supplied by milk and yoghurt. Magnesium can be obtained from green leafy vegetables such as spinach, parsley, turnip, radish, and beet tops. These vegetables should, preferably, be taken in salad form or should be lightly cooked.

Dietary Considerations

Diet plays an important role in building up health for gaining weight. Underweight persons should eat frequent small meals as they tend to feel full quickly. The weight-building quality of a food is measured by the number of calories it contains. To gain weight, the diet should include more calories than are used in daily activities so as to allow the excess to be stored as body fat. The allowance of 500 calories in excess of the daily average needs is estimated to provide for a weight gain of half a kilogram weekly. All refined foods such as products containing white flour and sugar should be avoided, as they destroy health.

Other Measures

Regular exercises like walking, dancing, yoga, meditation, and massage are also important as they serve as relaxants, reduce stress, and induce good sleep. *Yogasanas* which are especially helpful are *sarvangasana, halasana,* and *matsyasana.*

Urticaria

Nettle-Rash, Hives

Urticaria is a common disorder, characterised by formation of weals on the skin. The disease is also known as nettle-rash as the rash of urticaria resembles the sting of a nettle. The disease may be acute, chronic, or recurrent. It is considered to be an allergic reaction like hay fever and asthma.

Causes and Symptoms

Raised red and white patches appear on the skin. They are accompanied by burning, intense itching, and stinging. Rubbing and scratching usually aggravate the condition. The outbreak of urticaria is sudden and the disease may affect any part or the entire body. The eruptions may be as small as pin heads or as large as a rupee. The eruption may fade in a few minutes or an hour in one place, but may appear in another. Other symptoms which accompany hives are fever, digestive disturbances, and prostration. The disorder lasts from a day or two to a week. Recovery is rapid and complete, though recurring attacks may take place at varying intervals.

There are several causes of urticaria. It may result from digestive disorders like mechanical irritation in the digestive tract or toxaemia. It may be caused by drugs like aspirin, penicillin, quinine, ipecac, and so on. Certain foods often cause urticaria in susceptible individuals. These include strawberries, tomatoes, cucumber, mushrooms, oatmeal, wheat, nuts, fish, eggs, chocolate, cheese, butter, and sausages. The bites of bedbugs, wasps, bees, mosquitoes, flies, and certain kinds of caterpillars may produce the disease. It may also result from emotional excitement.

Remedies

Salt: The use of salt is beneficial in the treatment of urticaria when it is accompanied by digestive disorders. In such a condition, about twelve grams of salt should be dissolved in water and taken by the patient. The throat should be tickled to induce vomiting. This will give relief and help in curing eruptions.

Alum and Red Ochre: These two substances are considered valuable in urticaria. An equal quantity of alum and red ochre should be ground together and the powder rubbed on the weals.

Rose-Water and Vinegar: The use of rose-water in vinegar is useful when there is severe itching on the eruption. About 35 ml of rose water and 25 ml of vinegar should be mixed and the mixture applied locally to the affected part. This will give immediate relief.

Mint: This leafy vegetable has also been found useful in relieving itching in urticaria. About 7 gm of mint and 25 gm of brown sugar should be boiled together in about 175 ml of water and drunk. This will relieve the itching.

Turmeric: The use of turmeric is valuable in urticaria. The patient should take two teaspoons of turmeric powder mixed with a cup of water daily.

Rauwolfia: The herb rauwolfia is beneficial in relieving itching in urticaria. One gram of the powdered root can be taken with a cup of water daily.

Dietary Considerations

As urticaria usually has its origin in the gastro-intestinal tract, the best way to commence the treatment is to adopt an all-fruit diet for about five days. In this regimen, the patient should take three meals a day of fresh juicy fruits such as oranges, apples, pineapples, grapes, pears, peaches, and papayas. The patient should drink a copious amount of hot water.

After the all-fruit diet, the patient may embark upon a well-balanced diet consisting of seeds, nuts, grains, vegetables, and fruits. The emphasis should be on fresh fruits and raw vegetable salads. The patient should avoid tea, coffee, alcohol, all flesh foods, refined foods, and all foods which are difficult to digest. He should drink at least eight glasses of water daily between meals. A glass of water containing the juice of half a lemon may be taken one hour before each meal and also between meals.

The patient should spend two or three days on an all-fruit diet, at regular intervals. This will further cleanse the system of toxic matters and help recovery.

Other Measures

A warm-water enema should be used daily during the initial all-fruit diet to cleanse the bowels, and later, if necessary. The patient should avoid exposure to cold and cold water. Fresh air and sunlight are also essential for the treatment and the patient should frequently expose his body to the sun.

One of the most effective remedies for treating urticaria is a hot Epsom salts bath to be taken three times a week. This bath is prepared by dissolving one kilogram of commercial Epsom salts in an ordinary bath of hot water. The patient should remain immersed in the bath from ten to twenty minutes. He should cool off gradually and care should be taken not to catch a chill afterwards. No soap should be used with the Epsom salts bath, as this interferes with its beneficial effects.

Varicose Veins

Dilated Swollen Veins

Veins are thin-walled vessels through which the impure blood is carried back to the heart. They usually have valves which regulate the flow of blood towards the heart. Varicose veins are a condition in which veins become enlarged, dilated, or thickened. This condition can occur in any part of the body but generally appear in the legs.

Causes and Symptoms

The first sign of varicose veins is a swelling along the course of the veins. This may be followed by muscular cramps and a feeling of tiredness in the legs behind the knees. In some cases, the normal flow of blood towards the heart may be reversed when the patient is in an upright position. This results in veinous blood collecting in the lower part of the legs; the skin becomes purplish and pigmented, leading to what is known as varicose eczema or varicose ulcers. Both these conditions cause severe pain.

A varicose condition of the veins results from sluggish circulation due to various factors such as constipation, dietetic errors, lack of exercise, and smoking. Standing for long periods and wearing tight clothing can also lead to sluggish circulation. Pregnancy may cause varicose veins due to increased pressure in the pelvis and abdomen, which slows down the flow of blood from the lower extremities to the heart. Women usually suffer from this condition in the early years of child-bearing. Obesity can also cause varicose veins.

Remedies

Marigold: The herb marigold is valuable in varicose veins. A compress of this herb should be applied externally in the treatment of this disease. The flowers of this plant can also be applied externally over varicose ulcers with beneficial results, as they are an excellent remedy for inflamed or ulcerated conditions of the skin.

Vegetable Juices: Raw vegetable juices, especially carrot juice in combination with spinach juice, have proved beneficial in the treatment of this disease. The formula proportions considered helpful in this combination are 300 ml of carrot juice and 200 ml of spinach juice.

Nutrients: Certain nutrients, especially vitamins E and C have also been found effective in the treatment of this disease. The patient should take vitamin C in therapeutic doses upto 3,000 mg and vitamin E in therapeutic doses from 600 to 1,200 mg daily. This will relieve him of pain and leg cramps associated with varicose veins.

Dietary Considerations

For proper treatment of varicose veins, the patient should be put on a juice fast for four or five days in the beginning, or on an all-fruit diet for seven to ten days. Thereafter, the patient may gradually embark upon a well-balanced diet, with emphasis on grains, seeds, nuts, raw vegetables, and fresh fruits. All condiments, alcoholic drinks, coffee, strong tea, white flour products, white sugar and its products should be strictly avoided. A short fast or an all-fruit diet for two or three days may be undertaken every month, depending on the progress.

Other Measures

During the initial juice fast or an all-fruit diet, a warm-water enema should be administered daily to cleanse the bowels and measures should be taken to avoid constipation. An alternate hot and cold hip bath is very valuable and should be taken daily. The affected parts should be sprayed with cold water or cold packs should be applied to them. A mud pack may be applied at night and allowed to remain until morning. A hot Epsom salts bath is also very valuable and should be taken twice a week.

Sunbathing and deep breathing exercises are also helpful. Certain inverted yoga postures such as *viparitakarani, sarvangasana,* and *shirshasana* are beneficial in the treatment of varicose veins as they drain the blood from the legs and reduce pressure on the veins. They help to relax the muscles and allow the blood to flow freely in and out of the lower extremities. *Padmasana, gomukhasana, vajrasana,* and *shalabhasana* are also beneficial.

Warts

Superficial Growths on the Skin

Warts refer to hard growths on the skin. They are common both in children and adults. Warts are capable of spreading, but they are usually harmless. They often disappear spontaneously.

Causes and Symptoms

Warts come in various shapes and sizes and usually appear as rough elevations on the skin. These elevations appear more frequently on the fingers, elbows, knees, face, and scalp. Those that appear on the soles of the feet are called plantar warts. They are very painful and the sufferer is not able to walk properly.

The main cause of warts is a virus infection of the skin. Plantar warts on the soles are usually contracted in swimming pools. Constitutional factors, however, appear to be at the root of the trouble. These factors lead to some defects in the proper development of the skin surface in certain areas.

Remedies

Castor Oil: The use of castor oil is one of the most important home remedies for warts. This oil should be applied generously over the affected parts every night. The treatment should be continued for several months.

Figs: The milky juice of fresh figs is another valuable remedy. This juice should be extracted from the fresh, barely-ripe fruits and applied on the warts several times a day. The treatment should be continued for two weeks.

Potato: Raw potatoes are beneficial in the treatment of warts. They should be cut and rubbed on the affected area several times daily, for at least two weeks. This will bring about good results.

Onion: Onions are also valuable in warts. They are irritating to the skin and stimulate the circulation of the blood. Warts sometimes disappear when rubbed with cut onions.

Indian Squill: The herb Indian squill is useful in removing warts. A powder of the bulb of this herb should be applied locally over the affected area for beneficial results.

Dandelion: The herb dandelion is another valuable remedy for warts. The milk from the cut end of dandelion should be applied over the affected area two or three times daily.

Marigold: Marigold is another herb found beneficial in the treatment of warts. The juice of the leaves of this plant can be applied beneficially over warts. The sap from the stem has also been found beneficial in the removal of warts.

Cashewnut Oil: The oil extracted from the shell of the cashewnut is useful in warts as it is a strong irritant to the skin. It should be applied externally over the affected area in treating this condition.

Other Remedies: Certain other external applications over the affected parts have also proved beneficial in the treatment of warts. These include juices of papaya and pineapple, and chalk powder mixed with water.

Dietary Considerations

Simultaneous with home remedies, dietary measures can help in the treatment of warts. The patient should be kept on an all-fruit diet for about five days. During this period, he should take three meals a day of juicy fruits such as grapes, oranges, apples, pineapples, mangoes, pears, and papayas at five-hourly intervals. Thereafter he may adopt a well-balanced diet of natural foods consisting of seeds, nuts, grains, fruits, and vegetables. Further short periods of an all-fruit diet may be necessary at monthly intervals until the skin condition improves.

Other Measures

A warm-water enema may be taken to cleanse the bowels during menstruation.

Whooping Cough

Cough with a Whooping Sound

Whooping cough or pertussis, as it is called in medical parlance, is an infectious disease. It commonly affects infants during the first year of life, and children upto five years of age. In some cases children upto twelve years may also be affected. The disease can cause serious complications in the lungs.

Causes and Symptoms

The child develops a cold with a marked cough which becomes more severe and spasmodic after a few days. At the end of this spasm, the child gives a characteristic whoop. As the paroxysms of coughing increase, the disease becomes less infective. Vomiting, which is frequent, may lead to the bursting of small blood vessels in the nose or the conjunctiva of the eyes. The disease may last for several weeks. The serious complications of whooping cough are broncho-pneumonia and infection of the middle ear. Convulsions may also occur in severe cases.

Whooping cough is caused by the micro organisms *Bordetella pertussis* and *Bordetella parapertussis.* Of these, the first one gives rise to more severe infections. The disease is very infectious and spreads by droplet spray.

Remedies

Garlic: Garlic is one of the most effective remedies for whooping cough. The syrup of garlic should be given in doses of five drops to a teaspoon, two or three times a day, for treating this condition. It should be given more often if the coughing spells are frequent and violent.

Ginger: Ginger is another effective remedy for whooping cough. A teaspoon of fresh ginger juice, mixed with a cup of fenugreek decoction and honey to taste, is an excellent diaphoretic. The fenugreek decoction can be made by boiling one teaspoon of seeds in 250 ml of water till it is reduced to half.

Radish: A syrup prepared by mixing a teaspoon of fresh radish juice with an equal quantity of honey and a little rock salt, is beneficial in the treatment of this disease. It should be given thrice daily.

Almond Oil: Almond oil is valuable in whooping cough. Five drops of almond oil should be mixed with ten drops each of fresh white onion juice and ginger juice, and taken thrice daily for a fortnight. It will provide relief.

Calamus: The herb calamus is another valuable remedy for whooping cough. A pinch of the powder of the roasted herb should be given with a teaspoon of honey. Being antispasmodic, it prevents severe bouts of coughing. For smaller children, the dose must be proportionately smaller.

Dietary Considerations

At the beginning of the treatment, the child should be kept on orange juice and water for a few days. The child may be put on an all-fruit diet for a few more days after the more serious symptoms have cleared up.

Other Measures

Epsom salts baths will be beneficial during the initial juice and water fast. In case of constipation, a mild laxative, preferably castor oil, should be administered. This will also relieve the pain in the abdominal muscles, which are usually strained during the paroxysms of coughing. The patient should be protected against exposure to cold and moisture as they are likely to aggravate the condition.

Appendices

Indian Names of Herbs, Fruits & Vegetables

English	Hindi	Tamil	Telugu	Kannada	Oriya	Marathi	Bengali	Gujarati	Malayalam
Almond	Badam	Badam	Badam Kayi	Madami	Badama	Badam	Badam	Badam	Badam
Amaranth	Chaulai sag	Thandu keerai	Thota koora	Dantu	Neutiya	Math	Notya	Choli-ni bhaji	Cheera
Aniseed	Saunf	Shombu	Kuppi Sopu	Sompu	Mahurisop Somp	Mahurisop Somp	Muhuri	Anisi	Sombu
Arjuna (Indian)	Kahu	Marudu	Tellamadi	—	—	Anjan	Arjun	Arjuna-sadara	Vella-marutu
Asafoetida	Hing	Perun-gayam	Inguva	Hingu	Hingu	Hing	Hing	Hing	Perun-gayam
Babul	Kikar	Karu-velum	Nallatuma	Jali	—	Babhul	Babla	Baval	Babola
Bael Fruit	Bel	Bilwa pazham	Maredu pandu	Seema dalimbe	Bela	Bel	Bel	Bil	Vilavam pazham
Barley	Jau	Barli arisi	Barli biyyam	Barli	Jaba dhana	Jau	Job	Jau	Yavam
Belleric myroblan	Bahera	Akkam	Tadi	—	—	Bahera	Bahera	Bahera	Tusham
Black nightshade	Makoy	Manatta-kkali	Kamanchi	Ganike	—	Kamuni	Kakmachi	Piladu	Manitha-kkai

English									
Bloodwort	Rojmare	—	—	—	—	—	—	—	—
Butea	Palas	Palasu	Palasamu	—	—	Paras	Palas	Khakro	—
Calamus	Bach	Vasambu	Vasa	Bajegida	—	Vekhand	Bach	Gandhilovaj	Vashampe
Cassica	Amaltas	Konnei	Rela	Kalke	—	Bahava	Sonali	Garmula	Kritamalam
Castor oil	Arandi	Amanakku	Eramudapu	—	Jada	Erendi	Bhorenda	Erandio	Chittamanaku
Celery	Ajwan-ka-patta	Seemai sombu	Sima sombu	—	Juani patra	—	Pandhuri sag	Ajwana pan	Sellary
Chicory	Kasni	Chicory	Kasni	—	—	Kachani	Kasni	Gulsuchai	—
Drumstick	Saijan ki phalli	Muring-akkai	Muluga-kada	Nurgekay	Sajna	Shevaga	Sajna	Saragavo	Muringakai
Dry figs	Anjeer	Atipazham	Athi pallu	Anjura	Dimiri	Anjeer	Dumoor	Anjeer	Atti pazham
Fenugreek	Methi	Venthia	Menuh	Menthina	Methi	Methi	Methi	Methi	Uluva ila
Finger millet	Ragi	Kezh-varagu	Ragulu	Ragi	Mandia	Nachni	Madua	Bhav	Moothari
Goose foot	Bathua	—	—	Sakothind soppu	Bathua sag	Chandan bathua	Betosay	Chilni bhaji	—
Grape fruit	Chakora	—	—	—	—	Bedaana	Bilati batabi	Chakora	Mundiringa
Green figs	Anjeer	Athipazham	Athipallu	Anjura	Dimiri	Anjeer	Dumoor	Anjeer	Atti pazham
Henna	Mehndi	Marithondi Goranti	—	Mailanchi	Manjuati	Mehndi	Mehndi	Mehndi	Mailanchi

English	Hindi	Tamil	Telugu	Kannada	Oriya	Marathi	Bengali	Gujarati	Malayalam
Hogweed	Punar-nava	Mooka-rattai	Atikama-midi	Sanadika	–	Ghetuli	Punarnaba	Vaha-khafora	Tharizham
Holy basil	Tulsi	Thulasi	Thulasi	Vishnu tulsi	Tulasi	Tulshi	Tulsi	Tulsi	Trittavu
Indian aloe	Ghee kanwar	Chiruna-ttali	Chinnakata-banda	–	–	–	Ghrita	–	Kumari
Indian gooseberry	Amla	Nellikai	Usiri kai	Nellikai	Aanla	Anvia	Amlaki	Amla	Nellikai
Indian spikenard	Jata mánsi	Jata mashi	Jata manshi	–	–	Jata munshi	Jata mansi	Jata mansi	Jata manshi
Indian squill	Jungli piyaz	Nariven-gayam	Nakkava-lligadda	–	–	Rankanda	Jungli piyaz	Jungli piyaz	–
Jambul fruit	Jamun	Naga pazham	Neredu pandu	Neralai	Jammu koli	Jambhool	Kalajam	Jambu	Naga pazham
Jaundice berry	Ambar-baris	–	–	–	–	–	–	–	–
Jujube	Ber	Elantha-pazham	Regu pandu	Yelachi	Barakoli	Bor	–	Bor	Elantha pazham
Kidney beans	Rajmah	–	–	Huruli kayi	Barabati	Pharas been	–	Phanasi	–
Lemon balm	Bililotan	–	–	–	–	–	–	–	–

English									
Liquorice	Mulethi	Atma-dhuram	Yashtima-dhukam	Yashtima-dhukam	—	—	Jashimadhu	—	Iratima-dhuram
Long pepper	Ppli	Thippli	Tippili pippallu	Hippali hipplibali	Pippoli	Pmpli	Piplamore	Pipli	Tippali, Pippali
Margosa	Neem	Vepa	Vepa	Bevu	Limba	Nimba	Nim	Limbro	Vepa
Marjoram	Marwa	Marru	—	Maruga	—	—	Marru	—	Maruvamu
Musk melon	Khar-booja	Mulam pazham	Kharbooja	Kharbuz hannu	Tarbhuja	Kharbooja	Kharmuj	Kharbooja	—
Oat meal	Vilayati jau	–	Yavalu	—	—	Jav	Jai	Jav	—
Olive	Jatoon	—	—	—	—	—	—	—	—
Papaya	Papita	Pappali-kai	Boppaikai	Parangi	Amruta bhanda	Papaya	Pempe	Papayi	Omakaya
Pigeon Pea	Arhar dal	Tuvurum paruppu	Kandi pappu	Thugare bele	Harada	Tur dal	Arhar dal	Tuver	Tuvara parippu
Pomegranate	Anar	Mathalam pazham	Donima pandu	Dalimbari	Dalimba	Dalimb	Dalim	Dalamb	Mathalam pazham
Psoralea	Babchi	Karokari-shi	Kala gija			Babchi	Lata kasturi	Bavachi	—
Rauwolfia	Sarpaga-ndha	Chavanda avalpuri	Patala-ganthi			Harkaya	Chandra	—	Avlpori
Rhubarb	Revand-chini	Nattuire-yalchini	Nattuveva-lchini			Revatchini	Kokima	Gammire-vand chini	—

English	Hindi	Tamil	Telugu	Kannada	Oriya	Marathi	Bengali	Gujarati	Malayalam
Ribbed gourd	Torai	Pirrkankai	Beerd kayi	Heeraikar	Janchi	Dodka	Jhinga	Turia	Peechinga
Rosemary	Rusmari	—	—	—	—	—	—	—	—
Rough chaff	Chirchita	Nayuruvi	Uttarani	Uttaranee	—	Aghada	Apang	Safed agheda	Kadaladi
Snake gourd	Chachinda	Padava-langai	Pottakayi	Padavala	Chachinda	Padval	Chichinga	Pandola	Pandaval-anga
Spinach	Palak	Pasalai	Bachchali	—	Palanga	Palak	Palang	Palak	Vasala
Valerian	Jalakan	—	—	—	—	Kalavala	—	—	—
Watercress	Jalkumb	Alli illai	Aditayalu	Alvi	—	Ahliv	Chandrasana	Asalia	Thutta-kaya-kami-kai
Watermelon	Tarbooj	Darbusini	Puchakay	Kallangadi	Tarvuja	Kalingad	Tarmuj	Tarbuj	Thannir Muthari
Winter cherry	Asgand nagori	Amu-kkira	Vajigandha	Amangura	—	—	Asvagandha	—	Amukkiram
Wood apple	Bael	Narivilian	Velaga	—	—	—	Kathbel	—	—
Wormwood	Afsanthin	—	—	—	—	—	—	—	—
Zizyphus	Ber	Illandai	Gangarenu	Bore	Barakoli	Bor	Ber	Bor	Badram

Glossary

Albumin. Any of a class of water-soluble proteins found in egg-white, milk, blood, etc.

Allergen. Any substance that causes an allergic reaction.

Angina pectoris. Pain in the chest brought on by exertion, occuring due to an inadequate blood supply to the heart.

Anthelmintic. Any drug or agent used to destroy parasitic worms, especially intestinal ones.

Antigen. A foreign substance which causes the body to produce antibodies.

Antipyretic drug. A drug that reduces fever.

Asanas. Body postures adopted in Yoga.

Bronchiectasis. Dilatation of the bronchi, the air passages.

Caecum. A blind-ended pouch at the junction of the small and large intestines.

Calculus. A stone or stony mass of minerals formed within the body.

Camphor. A white, translucent, crystalline, swiftly-evaporating substance with an aromatic smell.

Cardiac ischaemia. A reduction of blood supply to the heart.

Carminative. A mixture of medicines which sharpens the appetite.

Cirrhosis. A chronic disease of the liver marked by the degeneration of cells and the thickening of surrounding tissues, as a result of alcoholism, hepatitis, etc.

Coronary thrombosis. A blockage of the blood flow caused by a blood in a coronary artery.

Cortisone. A steroid hormone produced by the outer part of the adrenal glands or synthetically, and used medicinally, especially against inflammation and allergy.

Decanted. Gradually poured from one container to another, without disturbing the sediment.

Decoction. A process of boiling down so as to extract some essence.

Denatured. A change of properties in a substance due to the effects of another substance being added.

Diaphoretic. An agent inducing perspiration.

Diaphoretic. That which induces perspiration.

Diuretic. Any substance causing an increased output of urine.

Emulsion. A fine dispersion of fatty liquid in another liquid, usually water.

Endocrine glands. Glands secreting directly into the blood stream—also known as ductless glands.

Endometrium. The membrane lining of the womb.

Endotoxin. A toxin produced inside certain bacteria.

Expectorant. A medication that facilitates the coughing out of phlegm, etc.

Expothalmic goitre. Overactivity of the thyroid gland, resulting in eyeballs protuding out.

Glutanic acid. A naturally occuring amino-acid, a constituent of many proteins.

Gonads. Testicles or ovaries.

Hydrotherapy. The use of water, generally in the form of exercises, in the treatment of disorders.

Hyperglycaemia. An excess of glucose in the blood stream.

Infarction. A small localised area of dead tissue caused by an inadequate blood supply.

Infusion. A liquid obtained by steeping the herb, etc. in liquid to extract the content.

Insulin. A hormone produced in the pancreas by the islets of Langherhans, regulating the amount of glucose in the blood and the lack of which causes diabetes.

Malic acid. An organic acid found in unripe apples and other fruits.

Melanin. A dark-brown to black pigment occuring in the hair, skin, and iris of the eye, that is responsible for tanning of the skin when exposed to the sunlight.

Mucilage. A sticky substance extracted from certain plants.

Myocardial infarction. Stoppage of blood supply to the heart muscle, resulting in its destruction.

Myrobalans. Dried fruits of the trees *amla, harad,* and *bahera.*

Myxoedema. A syndrome caused by hypothyroidism, resulting in thickening of the skin, weight gain, mental dullness, loss of energy and sensitivity to cold.

Oxalic acid. A mild and sour acid found in some fruits and herbs.

Pantothenic acid. A vitamin of the B complex group which is essential for the oxidation of fats and carbohydrates.

Parotid gland. A salivary gland in front of the ear.

Pestle. A club-shaped appliance used for pounding substances.

Phospholipids. Any lipid consisting of a phosphate group and one or more fatty acids.

Pituitary gland. A small ductless gland at the base of the brain secreting various hormones essential for growth and other bodily functions.

Poultice. A soft, medicated and usually heated mass applied to the body and kept in place with muslin, etc. for relieving soreness and inflammation.

Purine. A product of protein metabolism.

Pustule. A blister containing pus.

Rhizome. An underground rootlike stem bearing both roots and shoots.

Rubafacient. A counter irritant that stimulates the blood supply.

Scarlet fever. An infectious bacterial fever, which affects mainly children, giving them a scarlet rash.

Sebaceous glands. Glands secreting or conveying oily matter to lubricate the skin or hair.

Tannic acid. A complex natural organic compound of a yellowish colour used as an astringent.

Tannin. An astingent chemical substance found in tea, coffee, and the barks of some trees.

Tenesmus. A continual inclination to evacuate the bowels or bladder accompained by painful straining.

Thyroid gland. A large ductless gland in the neck secreting a hormone which regularises growth and development through the rate of metabolism.

Triglycerides. A kind of fat which exists in the blood.

Uraemia. A morbid condition due to the excessive presence of urinary matter in the blood.

Uric acid. A crystalline acid forming a constituent of urine.

Vesicle. A blister.

Warts. A small growth on the skin, usually caused by a virus.

Bibliography

Abdul, Hamed Saheb H. *The Complete Book of Home Remedies*. New Delhi: Orient Paperbacks, 1982.

Aman. *Medicinal Secrets of Your Food*. Mysore: Indo American Hospital, 1985.

Bakhru, H.K. *Foods That Heal*. New Delhi: Orient Paperbacks, 1991. *Herbs That Heal*. New Delhi: Orient Paperbacks, 1992.

Bricklen, Mark. *Rodale's Encyclopaedia of Natural Home Remedies*. 1st Indian Reprint. Bombay: D.B. Taraporevala & Sons Pvt. Ltd., 1986.

Charmine, Susan E. *The Complete Raw Juice Therapy*. Northamptonshire: Thorsons Publishing Group, 1977.

Chopra, R.N., I.C. Chopra, K.L. Handa & L.D. Kapur. *Indigenous Drugs of India*. Calcutta: Academic Publishers, 1982.

Clarke, Linda. *A Handbook of Natural Remedies for Common Ailments*. 1st ed. New York: Pocket Books, 1977.

Dastur, J.F. *Medicinal Plants of India and Pakistan*. Reprint. Bombay: D.B. Taraporevala & Co. Pvt. Ltd., 1985.

Khanna, Girija. *Herbal Remedies*. New Delhi: Vikas, 1986.

Lucas, Richard. *The Magic of Herbs in Daily Living*. New York: Parker Publishing House, 1972.

Mukherjee, K.R. *Protective Foods in Health and Disease*. 4th ed. Calcutta: Prakritick Chikitsalaya, 1983.

Murthy, Anjneya N., D.P. Pandey. *Ayurvedic Cure for Common Diseases*. 2nd ed. New Delhi: Orient Paperbacks, 1983.

Norris, P.E. *About Honey*. 4th ed. England: Thorsons Publishers Ltd., 1981.

Powell, Eric F.W. *Health from the Kitchen*. 2nd Reprint. England: Health Science Press, 1973.

Singh, S.J. *Food Remedies*. 4th ed. Lucknow: Nature Cure Council of Medical Research, 1982.

Verma, Ganpati Singh. *Miracles of Indian Herbs*. Third Reprint. New Delhi: Rasayan Pharmacy, 1982.

Miracles of Fruits. 9th ed. New Delhi: Rasayan Pharmacy, 1978.

Walker, N.W. *Raw Vegetable Juices*. 7th Reprint. New York: Jove Books, 1983.

Wesley, John. *Primitive Remedies*. California: Woodbridge Press Publishing Co., 1973.